Biomedical Sensing and Analysis

Iyad Obeid • Joseph Picone • Ivan Selesnick
Editors

Biomedical Sensing and Analysis

Signal Processing in Medicine and Biology

Springer

Editors
Iyad Obeid
Department of Electrical & Computer Engineering
Temple University
Philadelphia, PA, USA

Joseph Picone
Department of Electrical & Computer Engineering
Temple University
Philadelphia, PA, USA

Ivan Selesnick
Tandon School of Engineering
New York University
Brooklyn, NY, USA

ISBN 978-3-030-99382-5 ISBN 978-3-030-99383-2 (eBook)
https://doi.org/10.1007/978-3-030-99383-2

This Springer imprint is published by the registered company Springer Nature Switzerland AG
The registered company address is: Gewerbestrasse 11, 6330 Cham, Switzerland

Preface

This edited volume consists of the expanded versions of the exceptional papers presented at the 2020 IEEE Signal Processing in Medicine and Biology Symposium (IEEE SPMB) held at Temple University in Philadelphia, Pennsylvania, USA. IEEE SPMB promotes interdisciplinary papers across a wide range of topics, including analysis of biomedical signals and images, machine learning, data, and educational resources. The symposium was first held in 2011 at New York University Polytechnic (now known as NYU Tandon School of Engineering). Since 2014, it has been hosted by the Neural Engineering Data Consortium at Temple University as part of a broader mission to promote machine learning and big data applications in bioengineering. The symposium typically consists of 18 highly competitive full paper submissions that include oral presentations and 12–18 single-page abstracts that are presented as posters. Two plenary lectures are included—one focused on research and the other focused on emerging technology. The symposium provides a stimulating environment where multidisciplinary research in the life sciences is presented. More information about the symposium can be found at www.ieeespmb.org.

This volume consists of five chapters. These chapters all share common foundations in artificial intelligence, signal processing, and sensing. Most use some form of deep learning techniques to automatically extract information from electrical signals transduced from physical signals such as electroencephalograms (EEG). Deep learning continues to have a transformative impact on the signal processing field. Data plays a critical role in the development of such systems. Therefore, the Neural Engineering Data Consortium (NEDC) at Temple University, which sponsors this symposium, has a primary goal of promoting community interest in the development of big data resources. To learn more about these resources, please explore the NEDC web site (www.nedcdata.org).

The first chapter, titled "Restriction Synthesis and DNA Restriction Site Analysis Using Machine Learning," focuses a novel synthetic deoxyribonucleic acid (DNA) synthesis method known as Restriction Synthesis, which utilizes iterative restriction enzyme digest and sticky-end alignment to build a target DNA sequence from a reference DNA sequence. By synthesizing many genes from a well-curated generalized reference sequence using machine learning techniques, the efficacy and cost of Restriction Synthesis was improved.

The second chapter, titled "Human Detection and Biometric Authentication with Ambient Sensors," addresses the rapidly emerging area of smart ambient sensing and control, with a focus on elderly populations. A passive infrared (PIR) sensor was used to monitor physical motion and chest motion. The system is attractive for noncontact human monitoring because it is nonintrusive, inexpensive, passive, and relatively accurate. The chapter evaluates this technology in office and residential environments, demonstrating it is viable for human monitoring and authentication.

The third chapter, titled "Generalization of Deep Acoustic and NLP Models for Large-Scale Depression Screening," focuses on automatically screening patients for depression using voice. High performance is achieved using a combination of deep learning and transfer learning for acoustic modeling and transfer learning for natural language processing (NLP). The area under the curve (AUC) for a binary classification task is 0.79 and 0.83 for the acoustic and NLP models, respectively, demonstrating the feasibility of this approach for automated depression screening.

The fourth chapter, titled "TABS: Transformer Based Seizure Detection," introduces the use of transformers to predict seizure from EEG signals. The authors participated in the open-source Neureka™ 2020 Epilepsy Challenge. Transformers have had a dramatic impact on machine translation technology recent years but have not been as successful on physical signals such as EEGs. The authors use a neural network that includes fully connected layers, convolutional layers, and most notably a transformer layer. The system achieved a sensitivity of 9.03% and a false alarm rate of 31.21 per 24 h when evaluated using the Time-Aligned Event Scoring metric.

The fifth chapter, titled "Automated Pacing Artifact Removal from Electrocardiograms," focuses on the electrocardiogram (ECG) to evaluate the electrical activity of the heart for pacemaker applications. An automated method for elimination of pacing spike outliers in ECGs is proposed that uses modified Z-scores calculated from once differenced, detrended data to locate the pacing spike outliers if they exist. The process is effective at outlier elimination without distorting the physiological signal or affecting non-paced ECGs.

These papers are representative of the excellent work presented at this conference this year at a time when the community faced unprecedented challenges due to COVID-19. A sincere thanks goes to all our authors who helped make IEEE SPMB 2020 a great success. Due to COVID-19, this year's conference was conducted for the first time as a virtual conference. We had our largest and most diverse group of participants ever, with over 150 registrants. Papers, presentation slides, and videos are available from the IEEE SPMB conference web site (www.ieeespmb.org/2020).

Philadelphia, PA, USA — Iyad Obeid
Philadelphia, PA, USA — Joseph Picone
Brooklyn, NY, USA — Ivan Selesnick
December 2021

Contents

Restriction Synthesis and DNA Restriction Site Analysis Using Machine Learning

Ethan Jacob Moyer and Anup Das

1 Introduction

1.1 Problem

Restriction synthesis uses iterative restriction enzyme digest and sticky end alignment to catabolically synthesize a target DNA sequence. Typically, synthetic DNA synthesis is an anabolic process: subsequences of different lengths are combined one at a time to synthesize a target sequence. Conversely, restriction synthesis is a catabolic process as restriction enzymes cleave subsequences from a larger reference DNA sequence. Although there is an anabolic-catabolic difference between these two processes, both of them utilize subsequence monomers as an intermediate step to synthesize a target sequence. For instance, synthetic DNA synthesis relies on the anabolic building of single-stranded oligonucleotides, while restriction synthesis focuses on catabolically cutting out double-stranded subsequences from a reference sequence. In this way, restriction synthesis requires no such mechanism of oligonucleotide synthesis as is seen in synthetic DNA synthesis. Instead, it focuses on identifying subsequences by parsing through a reference sequence. Therefore, a generalized reference sequence must be well-curated before carrying out restriction

All source code is open-sourced at GitHub.

E. J. Moyer (✉)
School of Biomedical Engineering, Science, and Health Systems, Drexel University, Philadelphia, PA, USA
e-mail: ethan.jacob.moyer@drexel.edu; anup.das@drexel.edu

A. Das
College of Engineering, Drexel University, Philadelphia, PA, USA
https://www.drexel.edu

I. Obeid et al. (eds.), *Biomedical Sensing and Analysis*,
https://doi.org/10.1007/978-3-030-99383-2_1

synthesis such that only common subsequences that will contribute to the synthesis of target sequences are included. These are classified as applicable subsequences. Subsequences that do not satisfy this condition are labeled as inapplicable subsequences. Classifying subsequences based on this high-level criterion and observing how restrictions synthesis performs when using a curated generalized reference sequence is the main focus of this work.

1.2 Data Set

By following the synthesis of 1000 Mycobacterium tuberculosis structural genes during restriction synthesis, a data set of about 151,000 subsequences was obtained. These genes ranged from 1000 to 5000 base pairs and are from the National Center for Biotechnology Information (NCBI) [1]. Each subsequence had a class label as previously defined: applicable or inapplicable. These class labels correspond to which subsequences were (and were not) utilized in synthesizing each of the selected genes. The feature set of each subsequence was built using information from the gene of interest and the subsequence itself. In total, 16 feature groups led to 231 unique predictors in the data set. A subset of those 231 predictors is from a one-hot encoded vector of the nucleotides in each subsequence. Other features quantified the heterogeneity of nucleotide composition to gauge how likely a given subsequence is to appear at random. The remaining two predictors measured subsequence commonality and enzyme availability. These features described the relative usability of each subsequence in the restriction synthesis process.

1.3 Models and Experiments

Six popular techniques in machine learning were applied on this data set: support vector machine (SVM), random forest, naive bayes, k-nearest neighbor (KNN), artificial neural network, and convolutional neural network (CNN). The results of each model were compared using 10-fold cross-validation. First, different models were compared based on changes in hyper-parameter selection, and then the best models for each method were compared against one another. Using the best performing model, a generalized reference sequence was built from the classification results of unseen data and utilized in restriction synthesis. The results from the newly curated generalized reference sequence were compared to the that of the randomized reference sequence to determine whether there is a substantial improvement in synthesis efficacy and the cost of the synthesis method.

1.4 *Results*

The random forest ($n = 45$) model led in accuracy, recall, and F1-measure with the artificial neural network trailing closely behind. A generalized reference sequence was built from the subsequences that the random forest model classified as applicable. When comparing this newly curated generalized reference sequence to that of the randomized reference sequence in restriction synthesis, the reported percent yield of the target query sequence for a constant reference sequence size was far higher for the former. This indicates that the efficacy of restriction synthesis increases when using a well curated reference sequence. Additionally, the cost decreased when using this generalized reference sequence, supporting the adoption of machine learning in finding the most optimal reference sequence.

2 Background

2.1 *DNA Synthesis*

Since the 1860s, scientists have explored the biological make-up of DNA. DNA is a large biomolecule in the cell's nucleus composed of four chemical monomers called nucleotides, which are composed of a deoxyribose sugar, a phosphate group, and a nitrogenous base. These are known as adenine (A), thymine (T), cytosine (C), and guanine (G). The sequence of monomers in a DNA molecule serves as a code for constructing proteins out of amino acids at organelles called ribosomes [2]. For this reason, DNA is commonly regarded as the blueprint of life.

The field of molecular biology began with the isolation of nuclein by Johann Miescher in 1869. Nearly almost a century later in the 1950s, James Watson and Francis Crick postulated the process of semiconservative cellular DNA synthesis, which has long been understood as a trademark to biological studies [3, 4]. Over the past few decades, understanding this process has led to the discovery and development of many synthetic manufacturing methods, namely synthetic DNA synthesis processes such as oligonucleotide synthesis [5–7]. As a result, other areas of genomics have accumulated massive research interest allowing the field to advance at an incredible rate. From the start of the Human Genome Project in 1990 to the discovery of the Cluster Regularly Interspaced Palindromic Repeat (CRISPR) Cas9 system in bacteria during 2005, many researchers and scientists have attempted to fill in the gaps behind the molecule that is responsible for all living things on Earth. As science continues to explore these areas, the immense advancement in genomics technologies can be attributed to the growing reservoir of information pertaining to DNA research [8, 9]. Although humanity is on its way to adopting the full commercialization of advanced genomics technologies, the cost of synthetically synthesizing DNA remains as the field's largest determinant [10].

While cells can chemically synthesize DNA continuously through a process known as replication, it is increasingly difficult to synthesize long continuous sequences of DNA in vitro. For this reason, synthetic DNA synthesis often starts with a process known as oligonucleotide synthesis. Oligonucleotides are short single-stranded DNA molecules 13 to 25 base pairs in length [11]. These molecules are first built using a four-step cyclic process known as phosphoramidite synthesis, which adds one nucleotide onto a growing oligonucleotide chain attached to a solid support [5, 7]. After these oligonucleotides are built, they are specifically aligned to one another using complementary base pairing. Finally, an enzyme known as DNA polymerase is used in order to add nucleotides to any empty spots on the aligned molecule. Although this is a popular method for many biotechnology companies, it can be expensive ranging anywhere from $0.20 to $0.30 per base pair (bp) [12].

2.2 Restriction Synthesis: Theory

The rationale behind this work begins with the introduction of a computational model for a novel catabolic DNA synthesis method called restriction synthesis. Originally, the motivation behind this personal endeavor was to analyze the cost of this process as it was thought that it would be far less expensive compared to that of traditional methods. Restriction synthesis serializes the use of iterative restriction enzyme flanking in order to cleave, or cut out, subsequences out of a larger ambiguous sequence in the order by which they appear in a gene of interest. For simplicity, the ambiguous sequence is referred to as the reference sequence and the gene of interest is referred to as the query sequence. Figure 1 displays this process briefly.

The flanking process shown in Fig. 1 is carried out by coupling two simultaneous instances of restriction enzyme digests. Restriction enzyme digest is a typical laboratory procedure that utilizes a restriction enzyme and a linear or circular DNA sequence. The function of the restriction enzyme is to recognize a particular sequence in the DNA, which is characterized by the protein structure of the enzyme. Depending on the structure of the given restriction enzyme, it can perform either a highly specific or non-local predictable double or single stranded cut on the DNA sequence [13]. Figure 2 shows an example restriction enzyme digest using enzyme EcoR1 on a sequence containing subsequence GAATTC, and Fig. 3 shows a second example restriction digest using enzyme SmaI on a sequence contain subsequence CCCGGG. Both of these subsequences contain the restriction site for their respective enzyme. Each restriction enzyme may vary with respect to the relative position in their recognition site at which they cut the DNA sequence. In Fig. 2, EcoR1 cuts the primary (top) strand after the first nucleotide and the secondary (bottom) strand after the fifth nucleotide from the left-hand start site of its restriction site, while SmaI in Fig. 3 performs a cut after the third nucleotide from left on both the primary and secondary strands. The primary and secondary strand can also be identified by looking at the directionality of the sequence, or whether the sequence is running from 5 prime (5′) to 3 prime (3′) direction or vice versa. In molecular biology, this orientation refers to the directionality of the carbon backbone in DNA. While these two enzymes differ by their recognition sequence and cut sites, some restriction enzymes can be classified as isoschizomers, which are enzymes that recognize the same restriction site but may or may not perform identical cuts [14].

Once a subsequence has successfully been flanked out of the reference sequence, it is connected to the end of a growing query sequence using an enzyme known as DNA ligase. In the case of EcoR1, two sticky-ends are produced with equally long complimentary overhangs, while SmaI produces two blunt-ends. Typically, complementary sticky ends are much easier to ligate to one another compared to blunt-ends. This is because for sticky-ends ligation there is no ambiguity as to which side the two ends should be ligated. Conversely, blunt-ends provide no basis for DNA ligation as either end of a blunt-end DNA molecule looks chemically similar to that of a second incoming blunt-end DNA molecule [15].

Although there has been massive interest in synthetic DNA synthesis methods, no work has proposed a technique like restriction synthesis. With that being said, the idea of standardizing DNA subsequences is less novel but increasingly robust. In 2008, Dr. Thomas Knight and his colleagues attempted to standardize synthetic DNA subsequences by creating plasmids which can be targets for restriction enzyme flanking. Their idea was for each standardized DNA subsequence to have a highly specific biological function [16]. From this basis, they formed the BioBrick assembly standard, which is composed of roughly 2000 BioBrick standard DNA subsequences. Their aim for this work was to translate engineering principles to synthetic biology by allowing researchers to isolate and test unique genetic functions independent from the rest of the system. This is analogous to unit testing in systems engineering. Essentially, the group created an engineering framework for a linear system in genetic and molecular engineering. Their method of introducing these standard DNA subsequences was based around iterative restriction enzyme digest. Their two-step assembly process begins with flanking a standard DNA subsequence with restriction enzymes XbaI and SpeI and the BioBrick base vector with restriction enzyme NheI. The standard DNA subsequence is then inserted into the open region of the BioBrick base vector. These subsequences efficiently ligate to one another because all three restriction enzymes used in this process produce compatible sticky-ends. In short, the BioBricks standard is a process that "employs iterative restriction enzyme digestion and ligation reactions to assemble small basic parts into larger composite parts" [17].

The key difference between restriction synthesis and the BioBricks standard is that the latter only digests subsequences with the XbaI and SpeI restriction enzymes. Restriction synthesis relies on a data set of approximately 200 restriction enzymes from New England Biolabs [18]. In flanking a reference sequence with many restriction enzymes, restriction synthesis builds more composite subsequences homologous to those used in the BioBricks standard [16].

In restriction synthesis, the query sequence is the target of synthesis, and the reference sequence is the target of restriction digest. Although this relationship is well-defined, the ratio of the number of query sequences used for each reference sequence is not. There then are two extremes by which the reference sequence and query sequence are used in restriction synthesis. On one hand, there may exist a one-to-one correspondence between each unique query sequence and a unique reference sequence. In this case, each query sequence is synthesized from an independent unique reference sequence, which would require complete sequencing of all the components. Although this approach would result in incredibly accurate synthesis results, it would massively increase the cost of this method; the composition of each query sequence could be tailored to a specific unique reference sequence, but the synthesis and sequencing costs would eventually compound beyond its benefit. Therefore, this extreme case sacrifices cost for efficacy. On the other end, we can design one reference sequence from which many different query sequences can be synthesized. In this case, this reference sequence would be considered a generalized reference sequence because it is not designed for any one unique query sequence. This solution is a less expensive alternative to the former as only one reference sequence would need to be sequenced prior to restriction synthesis. There would most certainly be a decrease in the efficacy of the method when using a generalized reference sequence, but the cost would be far lower as it would require less sequencing. In this way, there is an inherit trade-off between the cost of restriction synthesis and its efficacy.

In order to optimize this second method, we have explored a procedure to carefully choose which subsequences should be included in the generalized reference sequence. By experimentally defining which subsequences fit specific criteria, we examined classification of DNA subsequences into two classes: applicable and inapplicable for inclusion in the generalized reference sequence. An applicable subsequence was defined as a subsequence containing a candidate fragment sequence, one that is common amongst different query sequences, that can be flanked perfectly by the combination of two restriction enzymes. The fragment sequence is the region that is of interest for the query sequence, and the subsequence contains that fragment sequence plus restriction enzyme recognition sites on either side of it. Additionally, the restriction enzymes utilized to perform this flanking must be commonly compatible with other restriction enzymes to support unambiguous sticky-end ligation. An inapplicable subsequence is one that does not follow these criteria.

2.3 Restriction Synthesis: Computational Model

We used a computational model to emulate restriction synthesis by incorporating an iterative restriction enzyme digest and sticky end alignment process. Through many simulations, we observed the classification results of different subsequences. A given subsequence must have satisfied three conditions in order for it to have been labeled as an applicable subsequence. These include a fragment match, an instance match, and a ligation match.

Given a query sequence and a reference sequence, the computational model simulates restriction synthesis by first searching for fragments that exist in the query sequence anywhere in the reference sequence. These matches are considered fragment matches. The length of these fragments varies with each search depending on which fragments are available in the reference sequence. It is more likely, for instance, to find a shorter fragment match than a longer fragment match at random. Each fragment search begins with searching for a large fragment sequence 16 bp long. The search continues by decreasing this value until a fragment match is found. Through this algorithm, each iteration for a fragment match ensures that the longest possible candidate subsequence is identified. If the algorithm reaches a minimum fragment match length of four bp, it will decide that there is no such fragment match in the reference sequence. If this occurs, the algorithm simply continues one bp position to the right and continues to search for the next 16 bp fragment sequence.

An instance match is based on whether two enzymes exist that can flank and digest the candidate subsequence. This condition is critical because while there exist many fragment matches, only a select few subsequences can be digested using restriction enzymes in the database. Using the restriction enzyme database from New England Biolabs, the simulation had access to 204 unique restriction enzymes and their respective restriction sites [18]. Despite the few number of enzymes, many of them have versatile recognition sequences, cutting a variety of DNA sites. Access to these versatile enzymes is one of the reasons why restriction synthesis can successfully complete on a variety of query sequences. All enzymes will be considered for each candidate subsequence. It should be noted as well that the process is able to use restriction enzymes from any database so long as they are formatted in a similar object structure. If the instance match criterion is not met for a given subsequence, the algorithm will start over and look for a fragment match one bp to the right.

In addition to a fragment match and an instance match, a third match is required: a ligation match. Some restriction enzymes cut DNA in a Z-like manner, where the product of the enzymatic digest contains nucleotide overhangs, commonly referred to as sticky-ends. Because many of the restriction enzymes create these sticky-ends on digested fragments, a ligation match is needed to ensure that sequential fragments are compatible. For instance, a subsequence that ends in an overhang of AGTA on the $5'$ end needs to be followed with an overhang that begins with TCAT on the $3'$ end. Also, some enzymes produce blunt-end fragments, or ends without any overhangs. These fragments need to be followed with other fragments that have these blunt-ends as well. This final end-to-end compatibility indicates whether a fragment sequence can be classified as a subsequence match and how the search process continues.

These three main conditions, a fragment match, instance match, and ligation match, dictate whether there exists a subsequence match in the reference sequence and whether the given subsequence is defined as applicable to be included in the generalized reference sequence. If it is, the fragment is extracted from the reference sequence and added to the growing query sequence.

Restriction synthesis was first implemented with the assumption that each fragment flanked from the reference sequence could be blunt-end ligated onto a growing query sequence. To standardize the subsequences that are flanked from the reference sequence, blunt-ends are created on both sides. Several enzymes, such as T4 DNA Polymerase, S1 Nuclease, Klenow, and DNA Polymerase, are used following the restriction enzyme digest in order to create blunt-ends from sticky-ends. Specifically, T4 DNA Polymerase to remove $3'$ overhangs, S1 Nuclease to remove $5'$ overhangs, Klenow to fill in $5'$ overhangs, and DNA Polymerase and an RNA primer to fill in $3'$ overhangs [15]. Because these additional steps and nonspecific ligation procedures are slower than that of conventional methods of ligation and DNA synthesis, further research must be undertaken to increase the rate at which blunt-ends can be ligated together. This manipulation of the subsequences allows for non-compatible sticky-ends to be ligated together without any loss of DNA. If non-compatible sticky-ends were ligated together, a DNA polymerase would add and delete nearby nucleotides randomly, which would alter the query sequence being synthesized. This method was changed so that only compatible restriction digests are included. This decreases the likelihood that any given random subsequence from the reference sequence could be used for synthesizing the query sequence. However, sticky-end ligation is known to be much more effective than blunt-end ligation because there is less side ambiguity due to alignment specificity. Furthermore, blunt-end restriction sites often lead to a phenomenon known as self-ligation, which is when one end of a subsequence ligates to its other end [19]. Taking the rate or probability of self-ligation into account will further complicate the model.

Previously, from 2017 to 2018 restriction synthesis relied on another assumption that the reference sequence from which query sequences are synthesized would be effectively generated at random. For this reason, the idea of a randomized reference sequence was coined. The model equation, $L = C * \frac{gns}{r}$, calculates the length, L, of the randomized reference sequence, where n is the length of the query sequence. This value must be large enough to account for all fragments found in the query sequence, and it also needs to be short enough to keep the price of sequencing low. Other constants, such as g, the complexity constant; C, the model constant; and r, the complexity rating were introduced and calculated using simple experiments. These variables allow the length of the randomized reference sequence to be estimated so that it is long enough to synthesize the entire strand and still be short enough to be cost effective for an experiment. Once this length L is calculated prior to synthesis, any sequence can be used in mutagenesis, or error-prone polymerase chain reaction (ep-PCR), as a basis to generate a randomized reference sequence of this length [20].

In previous computational models, a sequence containing $\lceil \frac{L}{n} \rceil$ repeats of the query sequence was used in the ep-PCR method, emulating a randomized reference sequence similar in composition to the query sequence of interest. The ep-PCR method assumes a 3.5% mutation rate because of a few assumptions. These include an increased concentration of Taq polymerase, an increased polymerase extension time, an increased concentration of magnesium chloride, and an increased concentration of dNTP substrates. Also, it is assumed that a dilution and pooling technique is used for about 64 cycles, or 16 dilution transfers, to avoid PCR saturation. With this degree of error for ep-PCR, 20 cycles can be used to still ensure a seemingly randomized reference sequence [21].

2.4 Related Work

This is a novel classification problem with many criteria. Many of which are not simply rooted directly the subsequence itself, such as the requirement for compatible sticky-ends. One group has previously explored the classification of longer bacterial DNA subsequences (about 500 bp in length) into their respective phylogenetic categories at the levels of phylum, class, order, family, and genus [22]. Models such as CNNs have been able to produce accuracies as high as 99.5% for classifying subsequences into their respective phyla. The accuracy is observed to decrease as the category becomes more granular with 67.6% for genus level classification. These results help to illustrate the various levels at which DNA can be classified. This group utilized a character-level one-hot encoding of their subsequences, resulting in a sparse representation of their feature vectors. Other works have used this representation in order to classify biological factors related to subsequences, such as their susceptibility to epigenetic changes like H3K9 acetylation [23]. Other applications of this DNA sequence encoding have seen accuracies as high as 96.23% for classifying subsequences as promoters, which are regions of DNA that initiate transcription. Because of the success of this method, we have adopted a similar one-hot encoding for representing our DNA subsequences.

Another group used a k-mer spectral representation to encode DNA subsequences [24]. By looking at the frequency of different short subsequences k bp in length (called k-mers) through a sliding window, a spectral representation can be formed that encodes the relative occurrence of k-mers existing in a larger sequence. In this case, the authors chose to abuse the "bag-of-words" model commonly seen in natural language processing. This DNA subsequence feature encoding method is computationally expensive as each k-mer has 4^k subsequences that can be included in the representation. Also, encoding DNA subsequences in this way requires that a representation be built from k-mers ranging from 1 to k nucleotides in length, leading to a sum of permutations.

Other groups have focused on fixed-length subsequence classification which limits the classifications to subsequences of the same length [25]. In our problem, this is incredibly limiting as not all applicable subsequences are the same size. For this reason, we added padding on our shorter subsequences in order to classify DNA subsequences of any length (see Sect. 3).

3 Feature Selection

The feature set of the data included 16 unique variables. Firstly, the SEQ feature is a vector of ordinal values corresponding to each nucleotide, where A, T, C, and G were assigned ordinal values 1, 2, 3, and 4, respectively, and the ambiguous base, N, was assigned an ordinal value of 0. This ambiguous base was observed when padding shorter subsequences since we are allowing them to be variable in length. After assigning ordinal values, one-hot encoding was used in order to form a sparse representation of the data. This increased the dimensionality of this feature five-fold. In this paper, we refer to the 215 values in the SEQ feature as the nucleotide features. These features most directly relates to whether a specific subsequence can be flanked by two enzymes due to the presence of restriction sites. What it does not capture, however, is the relative frequency of observing those sites and the prevalence of having two restriction enzymes to flank the subsequence. Including these nucleotide features in the data set is what motivated the use of a CNN. Typically, CNNs are for learning spatial relationships in data. The nucleotide features, in a way, serve as a spatial representation of the subsequence itself.

Another feature is LEN that encodes the length of each subsequence. Because each subsequence was padded, this information is lost in the nucleotide features. This feature is particularly important as it may serve as a simple heuristic for the likelihood that an enzyme could be used on the given subsequence. Considering that longer subsequences have a greater chance of containing restriction sites, this feature should show a clear positive relationship with the classification of the data. In preprocessing, this feature was normalized with respect to the maximum observed subsequence length in the data set.

Eight more features are obtained using Eq. 1. This equation describes the proportion of each nucleotide in a given subsequence. The first four are with respect to the subsequence itself, and the second four are with respect to the query sequence that restriction synthesis is attempting to build. These features are represented as $P(A)$, $P(T)$, $P(C)$, and $P(G)$ in either the subsequence or query sequence context. It was previously mentioned that ep-PCR was originally utilized to prepare a randomized reference sequence by purposefully mutating a sequence similar (if not identical) to the query sequence; these features were proposed as a simple metric to determine the degree of similarity between the two sequences.

The next four features are related to a novel sequence metric, the complexity rating, as shown by Eq. 2 and Eq. 3. These equations were used to accurately summarize the nucleotide composition of all four nucleotides with a continuous value ranging from 0 exclusive to 1 inclusive. Equation 2 is responsible for determining the deviation of an entire sequence from an equal nucleotide composition, whereas Eq. 3 segments a sequence based on preset values ranging from b to p and examines this deviation for each segment proportionally. In other words, the rationale behind Eq. 3 was to sum complexity ratings from Eq. 2 in proportion to the relative occurrence of k-mers size i in sequence size n.

Both of these ratings determine how far a sequence deviates from an equal nucleotide composition. A total of four features represents both the r_1 and r_2 values of a given subsequence and query sequence, respectively. This implementation of the complexity rating has a basis in the original model equation introduced in Sect. 2.3. The complexity rating, r, is scaled from zero to one in order to represent the complexity of a sequence. The composition of a sequence denotes whether a sequence is more uniform (has an r value closer to 0) or more complex (has an r value closer to 1). By rating a sequence's complexity, and ultimately its nucleotide composition, the metric identifies whether there exists long segments of repetitive nucleotides. An ideally random sequence has an equal ratio of all four nucleotides. This extreme is not biologically accurate as some sequences are AT rich and others are CG rich, but the complexity rating serves as a type of bookkeeping for a sequence's relative complexity (or uniformity).

Three different algorithms were explored to calculate r. The first algorithm, the complete calculation, assumes that the overall composition of the gene will provide a representative complexity rating for the gene. This is displayed in Eq. 2, where $\alpha = \{A, T, C, G\}$. It was discovered, however, that shorter segments within the gene could have repetitive sequences that would bias the complexity rating. As a result, a second algorithm was developed to correct this lack of specific consideration on short subsequences inside of the gene. The second method, the averaged calculation, first splits the gene into 4-mers and then averages together each of their r values. While this does solve the problem of misrepresenting a gene with short repetitive segments, it does not account for the other lengths of subsequences that maybe utilized in restriction synthesis. A third method attempts to weigh individually calculated r values by the relative occurrence of differently sized non-overlapping k-mers. The range of subsequence lengths that restriction synthesis takes into account are called parsing values. In an exhaustive search, the highest value for a given query sequence is $2^{\lfloor \log_2 n \rfloor}$, where n is the length of the query sequence. Subsequent values are calculated by recursively dividing the current value by two until it reaches a base value of four. This method calculates the r value for each parsing values and stores the number of occurrences of non-overlapping subsequences. The overall r is calculated using a weighted metric of each r with the number of occurrences recorded. This calculation of r is displayed in Eq. 3.

$$p(x, L) = \frac{occurrence\ of\ x}{L} \tag{1}$$

$$r_1(L) = 1 - \sum_{i \in \alpha} (\frac{1}{4} - p(i, L))^2 \tag{2}$$

$$r_2(n) = \sum_{i=b}^{p} \frac{\sum_{j=0}^{n-i} r_1(i) * \frac{i}{n}}{\sum_{k=b}^{p} \frac{k}{n}} \tag{3}$$

Lastly, two additional auxiliary features, C and EZY, were included to encode the commonality of a subsequence and the relative availability of each enzyme, respectively. The C feature represents the number of query sequences that contain the subsequence. This feature is analogous to the frequency of a term in a document in natural language processing. The EZY feature represents the number of available enzymes that can digest the given subsequence. These features were incorporated to gauge whether a particular subsequence is common in the data set and whether there are enough enzymes available to flank it. Just like the LEN feature, it is expected that there will be positive relationships with these two features as well. The notion for C is that when a particular subsequence is observed in many different query sequences, it will most likely be classified as an applicable subsequence. Similarly, when there is a greater number of enzymes available to digest a particular subsequence, there is a higher probability that two of those enzymes will be able to flank a given subsequence.

4 Data Selection and Prepossessing

Based on an initial raw data set of approximately two hundred million subsequences across almost one thousand restriction synthesis simulations, a corpus of 99,886 subsequences was selected with a 50/50 percent distribution between the two classes. Restriction synthesis simulations for the Mycobacterium tuberculosis Erdman strain urease structural subunit A gene (U33011.1_cds_AAC43473.1_1) were tracked using a randomized reference sequence 354,634 bp in length. This gene is 3800 bp in length. The resulting restriction map is shown in Fig. 4. With a randomized reference sequence of this size, the simulation was able to synthesize 79.87% of the query sequence on average. Even with this large, randomized reference sequence the model was still not able to synthesize the query sequence with 100% accuracy. This underlines one of the main motivations for the work: to increase the accuracy of restriction synthesis by using a well-curated generalized reference sequence. In one synthesis example, the simulation discovered 102 applicable subsequences out of a total of 33,050 candidate subsequences. For this reason, there is a huge, unbalanced class distribution within the data. Currently, the data is being classified under the assumption that these two classes are distributed equally. In reality, this would be impossible to assume because the discrepancy is too large. When this method was originally implemented, it was built with a cost analysis feature in order to gauge the relative cost when utilizing restriction enzymes in this way. Overall, the model calculated a price of only $0.0378 per base pair on average, which is considerably less than most standards [26]. This example should give some sense of scale to the second aim of this work: to decrease the cost of restriction synthesis by favoring the selection of long common subsequences in the generalized reference sequence.

During preprocessing, the subsequences were stratified into their respective classes to construct a 50/50 distribution. Then, the LEN, C, and EZY features were normalized according to their maximum value. The other features such as $P(A)$, $P(T)$, r_1, etc were not normalized as they are already inherently scaled from zero to one. Each of the nucleotide ordinal features were encoded using one-hot encoding where each nucleotide was assigned a vector of length five for the four nucleotides and the ambiguous base. After these preprocessing steps, the input data contained 231 features and a single target output. The data was separated into constant groups using 10-fold cross validation to validate each of the models.

5 Feature Analysis

Before analyzing class feature distributions, it is important to check for whether the features are strongly correlated with one another. In order to do this, a pairwise Pearson correlation between all non-nucleotide features was generated as shown in Table 2. Most of the features are either weakly positively or weakly negatively correlated with each other. This general weak correlation implies that the features in the data set are non-redundant and add different information to the prediction.

Next, the pairwise correlations between all nucleotide features were obtained in order to observe whether there is any nucleotide-nucleotide interaction. Because the table is so large, the data is simply summarized in Table 3 where each nucleotide feature is tabulated next to its highest correlated feature. This correlation test indicated high local nucleotide-nucleotide interaction within a subsequence. One would expect some degree of interaction due to the nature of restriction enzymes cutting at specific restriction sites. For most of the nucleotide features, we see that the highest correlated nucleotides tend to be those most adjacent to a given nucleotide.

As seen in Table 3, the maximum correlation per feature tends to drastically increase as the nucleotide feature number increases. This is because the nucleotide features farther from the start site at $Nuc1$ are more likely to be confounded with subsequence length. The first few features are the main site of the left-sided restriction digest for any subsequence, but the right-sided restriction digest is confounded on the last few features because the length of subsequences is variable. In other words, when examining the last few features of a shorter subsequence they may be confounding with the intermediate nucleotides of a longer subsequence when considering all of the nucleotide features at once.

In order to analyze nucleotide-nucleotide interaction further with less length confounding interactions, subsequences were stratified by length. Table 5 displays such a test where the correlation was obtained for only those sequences that are ten base pairs or less in length. From this table we can see that many of the sites have relatively low correlation, which indicates low local nucleotide-nucleotide interaction. While this might be strange at first due to the supposed nucleotide interactions within the constant restriction sites of a given restriction enzyme, it can be explained due to another confounding factor: the variety of restriction enzymes used. In fact, this low correlation implies that there must be many different restriction enzymes applied on these subsequences. Some of the most used restriction enzymes are those with shorter restriction sites composed of two to four nucleotides compared to a larger restriction site with eight or more nucleotides. This is due to the notion that shorter restriction sites are more likely to appear at random in any given subsequence. It then follows that this low nucleotide-nucleotide interaction displays that a variety of different restriction enzymes were utilized in this process.

As it was originally hypothesized, Fig. 5 supports that applicable subsequences tend to be longer on average. Not only does there appear to be a higher mean with applicable subsequences compared to inapplicable subsequences, but the right histogram also has a bimodal distribution whereas the left histogram has a unimodal distribution. In the case of inapplicable subsequences, if the lengths of particular subsequences appear at random it is easy to justify why there would only be one mode approximately halfway between the minimum and maximum observed length. However, a relatively apparent bimodal distribution for applicable subsequences identifies that two subsequence length categories are favored above all else. It may be that these two modes signify groups of subsequences that have more in common than just their lengths. This distribution is further supported by the high correlation between the $Output$ feature and the LEN feature noted earlier.

In Fig. 6, $P(C)$ and $P(G)$ are nearly identical for instances classified as applicable subsequences. This may indicate a high dependence between nucleotides cytosine and guanine within each subsequence. A similar trend is observed for $P(A)$ and $P(T)$. Since both of these pairs of distributions follow each other, it is not unlikely that the algorithm favors AT rich or CG rich subsequences. Although this is a naturally biologically occurring phenomena, the only way this could be incorporated into the data is if restriction synthesis favors applicable sequences when they are AT or CG rich. This may call for more features such as $P(AT)$ or $P(CG)$ to examine whether this relationship still holds.

Also, as seen in Fig. 7, the distribution of $P(C)$ for query sequences is nearly identical for instances classified as an applicable (left) and as inapplicable (right). This may indicate that at least for $P(C)$ this feature is not very deterministic of the classification of a subsequence. This may be the case for several reasons. The first of which may be due to the reliance of restriction enzymes on nucleotides other than cytosine. It might also be the case that cytosine at high proportion is included in some restriction sites but not those of enzymes most commonly used in restriction synthesis. For example, if restriction sites primarily include adenine, thymine, and guanine and not cytosine, then the distribution of $P(C)$ should be independent of the classification like it is observed here. It follows accordingly that we see changes in the distribution for the other three nucleotides when we stratify by the classification. In the case of these three nucleotide proportion distributions for the applicable classification, they appear more approximately normal than that of the inapplicable classification. This indicates that the recognition of these nucleotides in restriction sites is approximately normally distributed amongst all subsequences in each class.

Figure 8 shows that higher enzyme availability is more often observed with applicable subsequences compared to inapplicable subsequences. In the applicable subsequence case, the distribution quickly tappers off to the right side. The inapplicable subsequence distribution tappers off just as quickly to the right as well but there is a group of values between bin 0.33 and 0.36 that does not have any visible occurrences. Normally, the frequency of these missing occurrences could be explained by chance; however, due to the large number of instances examined in this analysis, this is not likely the case. One possible explanation is due to the existence of isoschizomers. If there are enough groups of restriction enzymes that recognize the same restriction site, they would always be accounted for by the commonality feature. For example, if there is some inapplicable subsequence A that can be digest by restriction enzyme Z that has five or more isoschizomers, it is very possible that all five of those isoschizomers would be counted when evaluating this feature for that subsequence. In this way, when calculating the proportion of enzymes that can digest any given subsequence, there is an all-or-nothing count for many of the isoschizomers depending on the sequence. Why is this not similarly observed for applicable subsequences? It could be that this distribution contains other subsequences that fall under the bin that would otherwise be ignored by the all-or-nothing isoschizomers restriction sites observed for inapplicable subsequences.

In the case of the commonality feature, C, Fig. 9 displays an unexpected relationship with the subsequence classifications. Upon initial consideration, one would have expected that the applicable subsequences would have a higher degree of similarity among a list of query sequences compared to inapplicable subsequences. A simple reason for why this is not the case is due to the distribution in subsequence length observed in Fig. 5. As applicable subsequences tend to have a distribution favoring higher lengths, it would follow that those longer subsequences would have less of a chance of appearing at random in another query sequence. Therefore, this can explain why there is not a high commonality among the applicable subsequences. Further it is important to note that restriction synthesis is not optimized to include the most common subsequences amongst query sequences. If this was the case, then we would expect to see this distribution for the applicable subsequences change dramatically with a noticeable shift to the right.

It is apparent in Fig. 10 that there is little to no difference between the subsequences classified as applicable and inapplicable for the distribution of the r_1 feature. When comparing Figs. 10 to 11, the latter has a thinner distribution compared to the former. This may indicate that the r_2 feature for subsequences has values more closely centered around a modal distribution compared to that of r_1. It is important to note that this distribution shape difference is also observed when comparing Figs. 12 and 13. Because the distribution of r_2 generally appears thinner than that of r_1, it may be characteristic of the r_2 feature to capture a tighter spread of values compared to the r_1 feature. One possible explanation is due to the difference in how each of these features are calculated. In Eq. 3, the r_1 feature is calculated over an entire sequence of length L, whereas r_2 in Eq. 2 is averaged across different lengths. The latter approach would introduce a tighter distribution.

6 Metrics

Since we are dealing with a binary classification problem, we can express our predictions with a confusion matrix as shown in Table 1. Specifically, we are interested in metrics such as accuracy, precision, recall, and the F1-measure. The equations for these metrics are expressed in Eq. 4-7 below.

$$accuracy = \frac{true\ positive + true\ negative}{true\ positive + true\ negative + false\ positive + false\ negative} \tag{4}$$

$$precision = \frac{true\ positive}{true\ positive + false\ positive} \tag{5}$$

$$recall = \frac{true\ positive}{true\ positive + false\ negative} \tag{6}$$

$$f1\ measure = \frac{2 * precision * recall}{precision + recall} \tag{7}$$

While the accuracy metric in Eq. 4 underscores how well a give model is able to predict classes correctly, precision displays its positive predictive value and recall displays its true positive rate. Often in machine learning, an increase in recall implies a trade-off with a decrease in precision and vice versa. For this reason, it is helpful to report the F1-measure which incorporates both metrics as shown in Eq. 7. In comparing each model, we would then favor those that score higher in accuracy and the F1-measure.

7 Methods

7.1 Support Vector Machine

SVM is a supervised learning model that creates a separating hyperplane between groups of data [27]. Given a set of training data and corresponding labels, the algorithm attempts to best categorize data by measuring the distance of each data point to the hyperplane [28]. By maximizing these distances, SVM creates highly reliable non-probabilistic classifications [29]. If the data is in N dimensions, the segregating hyperplane will be in $N - 1$ dimensions. A simple example is for data distributed across a two-dimensional (2D) plane. The hyperplane that separates the data will then be a single dimensional line.

While SVM models are powerful, they still require certain input parameters from the researcher that help to produce optimal classification results, such as the regularization parameter, class weight, kernel coefficient, etc. Although some data sets may not be linearly separable, kernel functions, such as the polymetric kernel, Gaussian kernel, and sigmoid kernel, may be used to categorize different types of data sets [30]. In addition to their versatility on different data classification patterns, SVM models are highly efficient in higher dimension feature space and when the number of samples is less than the dimension of the feature space. In the case of this research, this higher dimension feature space efficiency was one of the main reasons why SVM is used since there are a total of 231 input features.

7.2 Principal Component Analysis

In addition to the feature analysis, PCA was also used for feature reduction. PCA is an unsupervised learning method that reduces a feature space while retaining relationships in the data. By transforming a high dimensional feature space into a specified number of principal components (PCs), raw data can be summarized in a few dimensions [31].

7.3 Random Forest

Random forest is an ensemble learning model that implements a set number of decision trees based on subsets of training data for classification and regression [32]. A decision tree is represented by a tree graph with nodes and branches. Typically, each node is responsible for handling a subset of features, and each branch attempts to partition the data based on those features at the associated node. The goal of a decision trees is to implement enough nodes and branches to which data from the root of the tree can be partitioned down into pure classes at the leaves of the tree. However, as the maximum depth of the tree (the longest number of connected branches) increases, the tree becomes increasingly complex, so this metric is minimized when building a decision tree. Moreover, common operations called pruning and boosting to shorten or grow the tree, respectively. Random forest integrates a set number of decision trees into a model, so this is another hyper-parameter that needs to be specified by the user.

One of the features of random forest is its use of out-of-bag data [33]. At the construction of each tree, two-thirds of the data is included for training and the remaining one-third is set aside for validation after the training has completed [34]. During the training process, each decision tree is generated based on a segmented data set and a randomly selected feature set at each node of the tree [35]. When predicting based on new data, each tree provides a prediction, or a vote, for a certain class. The final classification for random forest is based on which classification has the most votes [32]. While a single decision tree may overfit data, many decision trees in random forest allow for the overfitting to average out between trees.

Some of the advantages of the random forest model include its high accuracy across data sets; its ability to process many features regardless if they contribute greatly to the output; its insensitivity to outliers, noisy or missing data; and its ability to form predictions using different variable types [36].

7.4 Naive Bayes

The naive Bayes is a probabilistic classifier that uses a strong independence assumption in order to assign classes to instances. The key assumption of the naive Bayes is that all of the features are perfectly independent of each other. In other words, given an instance x with feature set D, the probability of observing that instance in class C according to the apparently independent features in D can be expressed as $P(X = x \mid y = C) = \prod_{i=1}^{D} P(x_i \mid y = C)$. The model uses the following Bayesian rule: $P(C = i \mid X = x) = \frac{P(X=x|C=i)P(C=i)}{P(X=x)}$, where $P(X = x)$ is equal for all classes so it need not be included. Therefore, $f(x) = \arg\max_x P(X = x \mid C = i)\, P(C = i)$, finds the maximum posterior probability for any class i given example data x [37].

Often, the naive Bayes provides accurate classifications even if the features are not perfectly independent. This is because the predicted probabilities themselves need not be accurate with respect to the underlying probabilities. This is because of the fact that function f involves assigning C to x based on the arg max function, which is simply a comparison of two probabilities. If both of the calculated probabilities for two classes were calculated with the same changes to the equation (or using the incorrect assumptions) and if both are affected equally, then they can be compared to one another in order to perform a classification. This is the same reason why $P(X = x)$ can be removed from the denominator of the Bayesian rule that was initially expressed [38].

7.5 K-Nearest Neighbor

KNN is a simple supervised classification model that uses the distance between feature vectors in order to make a classification. Although this algorithm most commonly uses the Euclidean distance to measure distance, other metrics may be used such as the Jaccard Distance, Manhattan Distance, or cosine similarity. This model only has one hyper-parameter k, which is responsible for denoting the number neighbors to use to make a classification. It is often useful to set k to an odd value in order to avoid ambiguity.

The KNN model is first compiled with a training set. Then, a given test instance is compared to the k nearest neighbors based on feature vector distance alone. The given test instance will be assigned the class that is the majority for the k nearest neighbors. This follows independently for all test instances.

Unlike some of the other machine learning models, like naive Bayes, KNN makes no assumptions about the data and its features. Furthermore, another one of its strengths is that it is versatile as it can be used for classification and regression. KNN is not without its own drawbacks though. Because the model has to store all of the training data when making each classification in the testing set, it is highly memory intensive and computationally expensive. KNN is also sensitive to irrelevant features as it weights the distance of all features in the data equally. Lastly, because KNN is effectively dealing with high dimensional vectors when making comparisons, the model may be at fault to something known as the curse of dimensionality. As the dimension of the vector increases, the ratio of the minimum distance to the average distance approaches a value of one. This implies that as the dimension of the feature vector becomes large, KNN has a more difficult time forming accurate classifications. This is something we took into account when evaluating the KNN model since our feature vectors have 231 values each. A remedy to fix this is to simply implement feature selection and reduction before applying KNN to shrink the feature space [39].

7.6 Artificial Neural Network

ANN is a biologically inspired supervised learning model commonly represented by a directed, weighted graph with layers and units like in Fig. 18 [40]. The composition of an ANN includes an input layer, an output layer, and a specified number of hidden layers each with their own set number of units (analogous to neurons in the brain). While the dimensions of the input and output layer typically match that of the input feature vector and number of classes, respectively, the number of hidden units in each hidden layer is a hyper-parameter specified by the user. Typically, when an ANN contains one or more hidden layers it is considered a deep neural network (DNN).

Each unit in a given layer forms a connection with all other units in adjacent layers [41]. A connection implies that an output from one unit is sent as an input to the next unit. These connections are analogous to synapses in a biological neuron. More specifically, in the network all of the inputs to a given unit are individually weighted and then summed and sent through a (typically non-linear) activation function as an output to the neurons in the subsequent layer. Each unit has an associated weight that is used to adjust the impact on any given output. Thus, during any single prediction the signal from the input layer propagates through all of the subsequent layers. It is weighted and summed at each unit in the hidden layers until it reaches the final output layer in the network. These weights are one important factor for making accurate predictions. For this reason, the error observed in the output layer as a result of the initial propagation step is used in a second step known as back-propagation in order to adjust the weights in the previous layers. Different network architectures can be compiled with various error functions, or loss functions, which influence how the output error affects the weights of the network. Two frequently used error functions are the mean squared error (MSE) and mean absolute error (MAE). For instance, the MSE loss function tends to punish large differences in predictions, whereas MAE treats each error with equal weight. Often the choice of loss function is extremely dependent on the problem and the machine learning model.

The theory behind ANN models is that there exists some unknown function that maps an input space to an output space. Because of the interconnections in an ANN, it is able to form incredibly complex functions in order to best map an input space to the respective output space. By minimizing the error on the outputs, ANN models attempt to approach that unknown function to the best of their ability. In order to do this, ANN models are typically trained first with example instances so the network can learn the patterns based on data. After the ANN model has been trained with sample instances, it can be cross validated using a validation set of unseen data. If the composition of the validation set is not representative of the training set or vice versa then the model will perform poorly on the validation set. Moreover, if the model is trained on too many instances in the training set, then the ANN model will overfit that data and not be applicable on the validation set. One of the identifiers of overfitting is when the training accuracy is much higher than the validation accuracy.

As neural networks increase in size with a large number of layers and units at each layer, the complexity of the network tends to increase. A network with a lot of layers is considered to be deep, and a network with a lot of units at each layer is considered to be wide. When designing an ANN architecture, the user must pay attention to the selection of these hyper-parameters. A naive approach to selecting the number of hidden layers or the number of units at each layer is to perform a brute force of all candidate architectures. This would require a lot of time as the complexity to train an ANN model is incredibly high. Recently, there have been efforts to traverse and even search ANN architecture spaces in more efficient manners. One such approach utilizes binary search in simple binary classification problems in order to discover the most optimal number of hidden units in a single hidden layer for large input dimensions [42]. Another approach attempts to traverse a search space of architectures for the best k-complete architecture using an algorithm in $O(N)$ time instead of $O(N * M)$ time [43].

7.7 Convolutional Neural Network

A CNN model is a part of a class of DNN models that use a linear operation called convolution in at least one of their layers. The model usually begins with a convolutional layer that accepts a tensor as an input with dimensions based on the size of the data [44]. The second layer, or the first hidden layer, is formed by applying a kernel or filter that is a smaller matrix of weights over a receptive field, which is a small subspace of the inputs [45]. Kernels apply an inner product on the receptive field, effectively compressing the size of the input space [46]. As the kernel strides across the input space, the first hidden layer is computed based on the weights of the filter. As a result, the first hidden layer is a feature map formed from the kernel applied on the input space [44]. While the dimension of the kernel may be much smaller in size compared to the initial inputs of the convolution layer, the kernel must have the same depth of the input space. The inputs and convolution layer are often followed by rounds of activation, normalization, and pooling layers [46]. The last layer, however, is a fully connected layer where the final outputs or categorizations are determined based on how different features fall in line with the specific classes under study [45]. The convolution operation is commonly identified by the following two equations:

$$s(t) = \int x(a)w(t-a)da \tag{8}$$

$$s(t) = (x * w)(t) \tag{9}$$

Equation 8 explicitly denotes the equation for convolution, whereas Eq. 9 displays how an asterisk can be used to identify the linear operation. In both equations, x is referred to as the input. Typically, this is formatted as a multidimensional array, or a tensor, that matches the size and dimensions of the data. The second argument is w, representing a kernel, which stores parameters for the model also formatted as a tensor. This argument is adapted throughout the training process of the model. The output of both functions, s, is called the feature map of the convolutional layer. This is what is fed into the next layer of the network [47]. Figure 19 displays the proposed CNN for this data set.

CNN models are most commonly used for image recognition, video analysis, natural language processing, and time series forecasting [48–51]. Recently, CNN models have been utilized in areas of subsequence identification specifically for finding sequence motifs, which are DNA subsequence that code for transcription and enhance proteins in genes [52].

8 Results and Observations

Different hyper-parameters were explored in each experiment depending on the given machine learning model. For each model and model variation, the accuracy, precision, recall, and F1-measure were reported. The best performing model variations for each machine learning algorithm were found and used to make a final comparison between all of the methods. Each set of results were based on the averaged of 10-fold cross validation.

8.1 Support Vector Machine

For the SVM models, an analysis was completed with and without PCA. In general, there are a few main kernels that may be used when applying SVM such as the linear kernel, sigmoid kernel, radial basis function (RBF) kernel, and polymetric kernel. For experiments with and without PCA, these four main kernels were explored. Some sample plots were included in this work for when the classification can be visualized in two dimensions with two PCs.

SVM Without PCA The results of the SVM models are displayed in Table 6. The SVM model with a linear kernel resulted in an accuracy of 87.97%, a precision of 83.07%, a recall of 92.10%, and a F1-measure of 87.35%; the SVM model with a sigmoid kernel resulted in an accuracy of 79.00%, a precision of 77.90%, a recall of 79.65%, and a F1-measure of 78.76%; the SVM model with a RBF kernel resulted in an accuracy of 93.33%, a precision of 91.36%, a recall of 95.10%, and a F1-measure of 93.19%; and SVM model with a polymetric kernel resulted in an accuracy of 94.09%, a precision of 92.80%, a recall of 95.25%, and a F1-measure of 94.01%. As seen from the data, the polymetric kernel performed the best on this data set with the RBF kernel trailing closely behind.

SVM Without PCA When implementing PCA the number of PCs to which the data will be reduced also needs to be tuned. For this analysis, we explored the results of SVM when the data is reduced into two and three PCs for each of the four kernels. The results are summarized in Table 7. The results for these eight models were relatively variable. The RBF three PCs SVM model ranked the highest in terms of accuracy with 87.76%, recall with 93.27%, and the F1-measure with 86.93%, but the polymetric kernel two PCs SVM model ranked the highest in terms of precision with 82.79%. The overall best performing model was the RBF three PCs SVM model because of its high accuracy, recall, and F1-measure, which are arguably the most important metrics in this analysis. A possible interpretation for why the RBF generally performed the best is that it is able to form interpolations in the data above and below local extrema and it more rigorously fits to the known data compared to that of a polymetric or linear kernel [53].

When the data is reduced down to two PCs, the two classes are not easily distinguishable from one another with a clear decision boundary. This implies that the features are very similar to one another as PCA seemingly merges both classes together. Since most of the features are based on the nucleotides in each subsequence, it is possible that this is causing this observed low dimensional similarity. Specifically, of the 231 features included for classification, 215 of them are based on one-hot encoded nucleotide ordinal features. It is not difficult to find subsequences that are similar based on common short stretches of nucleotides shared between them. For instance, two 10-mers (10 nucleotide subsequences) may contain two sets of 2-mers in common at similar positions along their subsequences, yet these two 2-mers may play an important role in the restriction enzyme recognition on the ends of the subsequences. If we extrapolate this line of thought to every single similarity that may exist between subsequences, it is possible that they might cluster and even blend together as is observed. It is for this reason that very similar subsequences at that dimension of the data appears similar when in reality they belong to different classes. Now, when the data is summarized to only two PCs from 215 features that distinction is even more difficult to make. Although this blend between similar subsequences exists in the reduced two PCs data, PCA can still cluster most of each class together.

When applying the polymetric kernel, the degree of the polynomial must also be specified. The default value of this parameter in the package we used is three, indicating that the polynomial used in Fig. 17 is at most a cubic function. Because of the well-known trade-off between bias and variance in machine learning, we were careful with increasing this value further.

8.2 *Random Forest*

As previously mentioned, the random forest model has one hyper-parameter that specifies the number of decision trees to use when making a prediction on input data. In this work, we began with testing the random forest model with 10 to 50 trees in multiples of five (10, 15, ..., 45, 50). As shown in Table 8, the most optimal number of decision trees for random forest was 45 as that is when accuracy, precision, and the F1-measure are all at a maximum. Although the recall metric was observed to be a maximum at one other random forest hyper-parameter setting ($n = 50$), 45 decision trees appear to be the most optimal for this classification problem. Further inspection into the number of decision trees between the values of 40 and 50 might reveal slightly better results. Since the improvement of the metrics would appear to be on the magnitude of the hundredths, any other optimum is assumed to be just as good as the current best performing model. Therefore, this was the most optimal settings for random forest in the scope of this problem.

For this given random forest model, the results are displayed in Table 12. This model performed very well with an accuracy of 95.53%, a precision of 94.12%, a recall of 96.86%, and a F1-measure of 95.47%. This model is currently the best performing for this data set. This is still true when evaluating the other hyper-parameter settings for random forest explored in Table 8. Even with a relatively few number of decision trees ($n = 10$), the model still made accurate predictions. Thus, it follows that decision trees might be the most optimal classifier for this type of problem. It begs the question of why this model performs the best. If a collection of decision trees is able to easily model the relationships in the data, then there must be a subset of patterns that can be represented in a decision tree-like structure. This is because the basic building blocks of a decision tree are feature nodes with relatively simple decisions, such as whether a continuous feature is above or below a certain threshold. If we connect this underlying phenomenon to the performance of this model, we can hypothesize that the relationships that allow the random forest model to perform so well are relatively simple. In the scope of the feature set, a few simple decision rules might be according to the length of a subsequence since we have repeatedly seen a clear correlation with that feature relative to the applicability of a subsequence. Also, there might be some simple relationships in the nucleotide features as most of them seem to correlate highly with one another as observed in Table 3.

8.3 Naive Bayes

Unlike the other machine learning methods, naive Bayes classification does not have many typical hyper-parameters. Therefore, this section will not contain any hyper-parameter selection for this model. This model did not perform well when compared to the other methods. As shown in Table 12, the naive Bayes model resulted in an accuracy of 78.87%, a precision of 58.84%, a recall of 98.16%, and a F1-measure of 73.58%. This architecture performed the worst overall right behind KNN. Although KNN was the next best performing model, the jump in performance for all metrics except for recall is around 20 to 30%.

It is important to evaluate why the naive Bayes model performed so poorly compared to the other machine learning models. Like mentioned earlier in Sect. 7.4, naive Bayes assumes that each feature is independent from one another when determining the likelihood of a subsequence belonging to a class. This strong independence assumption might be the reason why this model performed so poorly. None of the other models assume this. On the other extreme, the ANN and CNN models actually incorporate layers that form dependencies between different features. As these models perform much better than naive Bayes and incorporate feature dependence, we can conclude that feature independence is what is causing this model to perform so poorly. Another reason why this might be the case is because of the structure of the data. One cannot simply look at the first nucleotide feature independently of the other nucleotide features since the recognition of different restriction enzymes is what majorly impacted the labels of this dataset.

8.4 K-Nearest Neighbor

KNN models rely on a single hyper-parameter k that denotes the number of nearest training instances when forming a prediction on an unseen test instance. The majority in the k nearest neighbors denote the model's prediction. Usually, k is chosen among a set of only odd integers in order to remove ambiguity in binary classification problems. If k was even, there could exist a tie when forming a classification for a given test instance. In other words, given an even integer k the test instance might have $k/2$-nearest neighbors that belong to one class and $k/2$-nearest neighbors that belong to the other. If this were to happen, the KNN model would randomly form a classification. Therefore, k is chosen to be strictly odd in order to avoid this.

In our case, KNN was applied with 10-fold cross validation on the 95,292 instances in the data set with k equal to 1, 3, 5, 7, 9, and 11. The results of this experiment are displayed in Table 9. Since the F1-measure monotonically decreases from when $k = 3$ to $k = 11$, higher odd integers of k need not be explored. The accuracy for the KNN model is the greatest when $k = 3$. This model performed well with an accuracy of 93.15%, a precision of 93.14%, a recall of 93.16%, and a F1-measure of 93.15. Although this is the best hyper-parameter choice for KNN, when $k = 1$ the model performed better in precision and recall with 93.21% and 92.81% respectively, which is just slightly above when $k = 3$. The F1-measure is the highest for this hyper-parameter value, supporting that this is the most optimal hyper-parameter. As seen from the data, this architecture was the fourth best performing machine model right ahead of the naive Bayes model.

This hyper-parameter selection for KNN confirms two points issued previously in the paper. First, when looking at the two PCs data distribution for the SVM classification it was noted that subsequences are highly similar and thus tend to cluster together despite their different class labels. This trend was also observed with the KNN hyper-parameter selection $k = 3$, indicating that only the most adjacent neighbors are required to form a prediction. Second, the KNN algorithm does not imply any interaction between features like ANN or DNN. Instead, it computes a distance based on the features independently of one another. As this KNN model simply uses the Euclidean distance measure, this can just be thought of as vector subtraction. KNN does not assume that these features are independent from one another like in the naive Bayes model because the total Euclidean distance considering all features is basically what determines the classification of a test instance relative to training instances. Instead, this algorithm relaxes some of the independence that was assumed in naive Bayes, yet not to the degree that is observed with ANN and CNN. As this model performs better than the naive Bayes model with more (but not complete) dependence among the features, this further indicates that feature dependence is necessary in order to form accurate predictions on this data set.

8.5 Artificial Neural Network (ANN)

There are many different hyper-parameters for ANN models such as the number of hidden layers, the number of units at each hidden layer, the learning rate, the activation function, etc. This paper proposes an eight-layered ANN model architecture with an input layer, output layer, and six hidden layers. Each hidden layer has half as many units as the previous layer. This model architecture can be simply summarized with the vector [231, 231, 115, 57, 28, 14, 7, 1], where each value in the vector denotes the number of units in each layer with the first value belonging to the input layer and the last value belonging to the output layer. The input layer is characterized by batch normalization, which is a method in neural network architecture design in order to re-scale and re-center input data [54]. After the initial input layer, the first hidden layer is marked by a rectified linear unit (ReLU) activation function, which scales negative outputs to zero and leaves positive outputs untouched. The next five hidden layers contain linear activation functions. Finally, the last layer of the network is the output layer with a single unit and a sigmoid activation function. The model is compiled with binary cross entropy and model optimizer Adam from Keras [55]. The ANN model architecture is displayed graphically in Fig. 18.

For this given ANN model architecture, the results are displayed in Table 10. The feature set is split into two groups: all features and only nucleotide features. As explained in Sect. 8.6, this is introduced in order to determine whether only using nucleotide features is sufficient for this classification problem. As shown in Table 10, when trained on all of the features, this ANN model performed well with an accuracy of 95.20%, a precision of 95.41%, a recall of 95.01%, and a F1-measure of 95.21%. When only the nucleotide features are used to perform the classification, the model results in an accuracy of 95.08%, a precision of 94.92%, a recall of 95.24%, and a F1-measure of 95.07%. Even though the non-nucleotide features are removed, the ANN model is still able to make accurate predictions on the data. In the case of recall, the nucleotide only feature model for ANN performed better than the all-feature ANN with 92.54%. As seen from the data in Table 12, this architecture is the second-best performing model falling right behind random forest.

8.6 Convolutional Neural Network (CNN)

CNN models have hyper-parameters similar to ANN models. Because CNN models contain layers with the convolution operation displayed in Eq. 9, they have a few more hyper-parameters including the number of filters, the kernel size, the stride, etc. Moreover, depending on the input data, the convolution operation can be applied at different dimensions. In this case, we are concerned with one-dimensional (1-D) convolution as the input is a single vector. There are other cases in which two-dimensional (2-D) or even three-dimensional (3-D) convolution is necessary such as in 2-D and 3-D image processing, respectively. This work proposes a 12-layered CNN model architecture with an input layer, output layer and ten hidden layers. This model architecture can be simply summarized with the vector [231, 231, 115, 115, 57, 57, 28, 28, 14, 14, 7, 1], where each value in the vector denotes the number of units in each layer with the first value belonging to the input layer and the last value belonging to the output layer. Unlike the proposed ANN model architecture, this CNN model architecture begins with a 1-D convolution input layer formatted to the size of the input vector. This layer is marked by a kernel size of three and a number of filters equal to the length of the input layer. Following this first layer of the network, the model continues with a 1-D maximum pooling layer with a pool size of two and similar padding. The next eight layers are composed of four sets of these two layers; however, similar to the ANN model architecture, each successive 1-D convolution layer has half the number of filters as the previous layer. After these rounds of 1-D convolution and 1-D maximum pooling layers, the model finishes off with a flatten layer that compresses the data into a single vector equal to the size of the previous layer and a dense one-unit output layer with a sigmoid activation function. The model is compiled with binary cross entropy and model optimizer Adam from Keras. The CNN model architecture is displayed graphically in Fig. 19.

For this given CNN model architecture, the results are displayed in Table 11. This model performed extremely well with an accuracy of 94.80%, a precision of 94.25%, a recall of 95.32%, and a F1-measure of 94.77%. This is the third best performing model right behind the ANN model.

Convolution was introduced in order to recognize local and non-local nucleotide-nucleotide interactions in the subsequences. Based off of the results, the convolution operation is not most appropriate for forming classifications as an ANN model with linear dense connections performed slightly better. Since CNN models are typically applied on pattern recognition and financial time-series where the features have either purely spatial or temporal relationship to one another, the CNN model is re-evaluated on only the nucleotide features [56, 57]. In this way, we are removing any confounding affects that exist between the nucleotide features and the non-nucleotide features when applying the convolution operation. The results for this test are shown in Table 11. This model performed well with an accuracy of 94.90%, a precision of 94.77%, a recall of 95.02%, and a F1-measure of 94.89%. By removing the non-nucleotide features, the CNN is able to better classify the data in terms of accuracy, precision, and F1-measure. In reality, this implies that those excess features need not be calculated because simply examining the subsequences themselves provide more accurate results.

It would appear that the inclusion of the non-nucleotide features actually slightly increased the performance of the CNN model with respect to precision. This implies that when all features are utilized, the CNN model classified some of the false positives from the nucleotide-only CNN model. There is no further explanation for why the accuracy, recall, the F1-measure were higher for the nucleotide-only CNN model other than these additional non-nucleotide features confound the relationships important to the CNN model architecture. Regardless, as seen by this data there is truth to the original motivation for exploring the nucleotide-only feature CNN model. The nucleotide-only CNN model performed the best overall for this category of machine learning models. Even though the all-feature CNN model did not perform better than the nucleotide-only CNN model, this model was still able to classify the instances accurately.

8.7 Model Comparison

Table 12 tabulates the best performing model hyper-parameter settings for each of the machine learning methods explored in this work. Overall, random forest ($n = 45$) performed the best in accuracy, recall, and F1-measure with 95.53%, 96.86%, and 95.47%, respectively. The all-feature ANN model performed the best in precision with 95.41%. Using this best performing model, we tackled the initially presented problem of this work: classifying subsequences for their inclusion in a generalized reference sequence. Specific metrics of restriction synthesis were compared when using the previously adapted randomized reference sequence and this newly curated generalized reference sequence.

9 Application

Before we explore the application of these machine learning models on the initially presented problem, it is important to understand how the cost and efficacy of restriction synthesis depends on the length of the randomized reference sequence first. Cost is measured in dollars per bp (relative to the query sequence under question) and efficacy is measured in the percent yield of the query sequence. When efficacy is measured in this way, we can determine for any given reference sequence length how much of a given query sequence can we expect to synthesize. Also, it gives us insight into the marginal increase in synthesis when increasing the length of the reference sequence by a fixed amount. While cost is thought to remain constant over range of reference sequence lengths, the efficacy is hypothesized to be proportional to the length of reference sequence. Another important metric to keep in mind is the number of applicable subsequences identified. For the restriction synthesis of a fixed query sequence length, a fewer number of applicable subsequences implies that on average each subsequence will be longer. The opposite is true for a greater number of applicable subsequences. When subsequences become too short, ligation between them becomes difficult. Therefore, we favor relatively longer subsequences on average and thus a fewer number of applicable subsequences. The number of applicable subsequences identified is then thought to decrease when increasing the reference sequence length. This third metric can also be used to explain some of the other phenomena in the paper.

Figure 20 displays the trend of variable lengths of the reference sequence with the number of applicable subsequences for each synthesis. As we thought, there is an inverse relationship between these two variables. The number of applicable subsequences for the longest reference sequence is half of that for the shortest reference sequence. When the reference sequence decreases in length, there are fewer total subsequences that can be utilized for restriction synthesis and the probability of observing a longer subsequence match decreases. Because the restriction synthesis method is implemented without replacement and the previously mentioned trends, this relationship is marked by a parabolic decline instead of a strictly inversely linear relationship. Therefore, the results in Fig. 20 are not surprising. When a longer reference sequence is used, there is a greater chance of encountering subsequence matches at random.

When paying attention to the scale of the y-axis in Fig. 21, it becomes clear that the cost of synthesis is generally stable between \$0.040/bp and \$0.032/bp. Although this 0.8 cent/bp difference is considered negligibly small, there does appear to be a decrease in price as the length of the reference sequence increases. This is unexpected because the restriction synthesis simulation is not necessarily designed to use the least expensive restriction enzymes when performing flanking digests. Instead, it simply chooses the first possible restriction enzyme to do the cut. One thought is that since the number of applicable subsequences is observed to decrease with increasing reference sequence length in Fig. 20, there are less enzymes required on average. This would explain the observed decrease in price. On the other hand, the number of applicable subsequences (and the number of enzymes required) nearly doubles when comparing the longest reference sequence to the shortest reference sequence, but the cost only changes by 0.2 cents/bp. As a result, there must be some other phenomena at play here that explains this change in cost.

The data in Fig. 22 is what we are most interested in. Even with the longest reference sequence of over 350,000 bp, the recorded percent yield is around 80%. As the reference sequence length decreases, the percent yield hovers around this value until it drops off below 70% at a reference sequence length of about 50,000. This figure further indicates that in order to reach a percent yield closer to 100%, the length of the reference sequence would need to increase dramatically as this distribution appears to plateau with an increase in length.

In order to further explore the given problem at hand, we must first compile a data set to give the trained model. The current length of the randomized reference sequence is 354,634 base pairs. Based on the feature analysis, the length feature of the applicable subsequences in the complete data set of 95,292 instances is distributed bimodally at 0.5 and 0.6. Since this length feature is obtained by dividing the length of each subsequence by the maximum subsequence length in the data set, we can multiply these calculated features by the maximum subsequence length in order to obtain the nominal distribution of lengths. For the data set used in this study, the maximum subsequence length is 43 base pairs. This implies that most of the subsequences are approximately between 21 ($21.5 = 0.5 * 43$) and 25 ($25.8 = 0.6 * 43$) base pairs long. Thus, in order to build a generalized reference sequence equal in size to the randomized reference sequence, we need on average between 16,887 ($16,887.3 = 354,634/21$) and 14,185 ($14,185.4 = 354,634/25$) applicable subsequences and just as many inapplicable subsequences for the classification. We compile a new data set of 78,930 instances with a 50/50 class distribution from the restriction synthesis of general Mycobacterium avium genes ranging from 1000 to 5000 bp.

Using the random forest ($n = 45$) model, we built a generalized reference sequence based on its classifications from unseen data. After the random forest model was trained on the entirety of the 99,886 instances that is used for 10-fold cross validation, the 80,158 instances in the new unseen data set were fed into the model. The classification of this new data set resulted in an accuracy of 90.62%, a precision of 86.74%, a recall of 94.05%, and an F1-measure of 90.25%. The decrease in performance compared to what is shown in Table 8 can be attributed to the fact that this model was trained on an entirely different species of Mycobacterium. Since we already know how well the model classifies on Mycobacterium tuberculosis from the 10-fold cross validation in each section of this paper, it makes more sense to evaluate the model on less related subsequences. Despite this shift in species, the data from this test suggests that sequence data can be partially generalized across related species. More tests would need to be conducted in order to determine whether this problem is species specific.

As a result of this model classification, 36,964 subsequences were predicted to be applicable for restriction synthesis. When compiled together this created a generalized reference sequence 1,010,226 base pairs in length. From this sequence we created one generalized reference sequence 354,634 base pairs in length and followed its efficacy and cost. In a way, this generalized reference sequence was compiled from subsequences of Mycobacterium avium genes. For this next experiment, we used this generalized reference sequence in the restriction synthesis of Mycobacterium tuberculosis Erdman strain urease structural subunit A. We do this for two reasons. First, we want to control the variability between synthesizing different genes so that we can directly compare these results to those conducted with a randomized reference sequence. Second, we want to note species-specific behavior.

When using the newly curated generalized reference sequence, we see that it performed much better than the randomized reference sequence in terms of the number of applicable subsequences in Fig. 23. More specifically, there are far fewer applicable subsequences on average for the most extreme cases on the left side of this graph compared to Fig. 20. The difference appears to be around 40 fewer applicable subsequences. Even on the right side of the graph the distribution dives below 100 and closer to 90 applicable subsequences whereas that of Fig. 20 never dipped below 100.

In examining the difference in accuracy, Fig. 25 displays that restriction synthesis with the generalized reference sequence hovers around 80% up to sequences as short as 150,000 base pairs. This is truly incredible since when using the randomized reference sequence, Fig. 22 shows that the method was truly never able to cross 80%. A similar note can be made about the other extreme on the left side of both graphs where the minimum is about one and half times higher in Fig. 25 compared to that of Fig. 22. Overall, by curating subsequences from a randomized reference sequence and creating a generalized reference sequence, the accuracy distribution shifted upward as a whole. Also, if the data were extrapolated to higher reference sequence lengths, the generalized reference sequence distribution for this metric does not appear to plateau as quickly as does that of the randomized reference sequence in Fig. 22. Instead, it appears to further increase. This is a good identifier that restriction synthesis is able to provide a much higher percent yield when a longer generalized reference subsequence is used.

The new cost trend in Fig. 24 does not have a trivial pattern. In implementing this new generalized reference sequence, it appears that the cost shifts upwards instead of downwards despite the overall decrease in the number of applicable subsequences. One would have thought that this increase would imply that the applicable subsequences would be shorter on average and thus allow the cost to be lower as less enzymes would be required. It could be that the most popular applicable subsequences require more expensive restriction enzymes than some uncommon applicable subsequences. A deeper cost analysis is needed in order to evaluate what exactly is at play here. Moreover, if this is true, then the restriction synthesis algorithm could be altered to favor the least expensive restriction enzymes available. This implementation would need to be compared for both the randomized reference sequence and the generalized reference sequence.

10 Discussion

Overall, the comparison between a randomized reference sequence and a generalized reference sequence displays that machine learning curated sequences will allow for restriction synthesis to perform with a higher percent yield for a given reference sequence length. This can be partially explained by the distribution in applicable subsequences that is observed in this work. It is presently unclear why the cost is slightly higher for the randomized reference sequence compared to that of the generalized reference sequence. As it was previously mentioned, a simple fix may just be to prioritize the least expensive restriction enzymes for any given cut.

There are a few details that should be addressed in the future work of this project. Only five nucleotides were considered with encoding them into ordinal vectors: the four nitrogenous bases (A, T, C, G) and an ambiguous base (N). This can be further generalized by adding more ordinal values for partially ambiguous bases. For instance, restriction enzyme AvaI has recognition site CYCGRG. The letters Y and R pyrimidines (C and T) and purines (A and G), respectively. There are several other letters for these partially ambiguous bases. Since they appear frequently in restriction enzymes, it would make sense to add them as possible ordinal values for the nucleotide features in future work. Although these partially ambiguous bases do not appear in genes themselves, they may add essential features if the subsequences are encoded differently. Subsequence regions can be broken down into the fragment included in the query sequence and the flanking regions that the restriction enzymes recognize on either side of it. A simple implementation could be to only encode these partially ambiguous bases in the flanking region and encode the fragment region with only the four nitrogenous base ordinal vectors. In this way, subsequences can be annotated with other features. For instance, two other features could be included to identify the positions along the subsequence that break up the subsequence into three regions: the left flanking site, the intermediate fragment, and the right flanking site. This would only be possible if the mapping for each enzyme on the generalized reference sequence was determined and stored ahead of time. Then, it would be less important for the model to identify fragment matches. This problem definition may change the results entirely.

One of the major assumptions of this work is that the two subsequence classes are equally distributed among the data. Realizing this is a strong assumption to hold for any machine learning problem, we would like to include relaxing this assumption in a future work. The methods explored in this paper cannot be applied on independent restriction synthesis simulations until this assumption is relaxed. As this paper attempts to address the applications of analyzing and classifying these different subsequences, it is imperative to explore how different models can be implemented that are specifically designed for unbalanced data. In our case, there are far more inapplicable subsequences than there are applicable subsequences as shown in an earlier example restriction synthesis simulation.

Identifying a way to efficiently relax this assumption is ideal for another reason in particular. While the nucleotide features of the data are easy to obtain through generating sample subsequences, the non-nucleotide features require context measurements from restriction synthesis itself. With this in mind, we observe in Tables 10 and 11 that when only the nucleotide features are used, they perform almost as well as when all features are included in the prediction. Therefore, it begs the question of whether these non-nucleotide features are needed at all. If it is determined that they are not, then generating sample test data would be much easier. This would be the real power in this model, because then the curation of the generalized reference sequence would be entirely independent from any simulations of restriction synthesis. This relies heavily on accurately representing the class distribution of the data. In the future, this can be mathematically estimated by identifying permutations of restriction enzyme recognition for random subsequences. Second, in order to implement this, we would need to strongly assume that the generalized reference sequence is species independent, which was only briefly explored in this work. Regardless, there are many future directions to improve the preliminary work explored in this paper and to satisfy more scenarios of restriction synthesis.

Appendix: Tables and Figures

See Figs. 1, 2, 3, 4, 5, 6, 7, 8, 9, 10, 11, 12, 13, 14, 15, 16, 17, 18, 19, 20, 21, 22, 23, 24, 25 and Tables 1, 2, 3, 4, 5, 6, 7, 8, 9, 10, 11, 12.

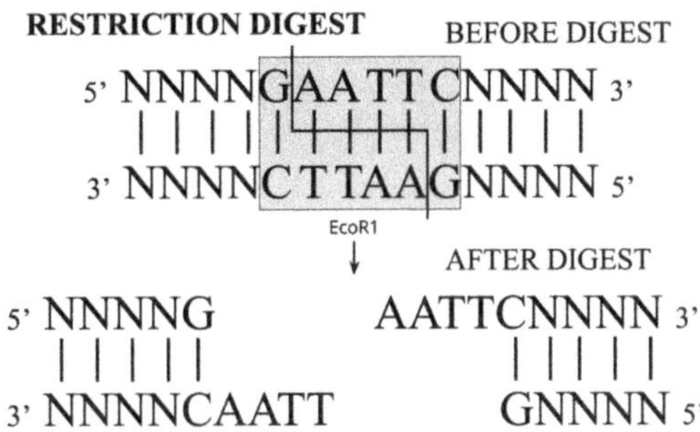

Fig. 1 Restriction enzyme digest of GAATTC using EcorR1 producing two sticky-end overhangs. In general, DNA is represented as a permutation of the four nucleotides [adenine (A), thymine (T), cytosine (C), guanine (G)] and an ambiguous base (N)

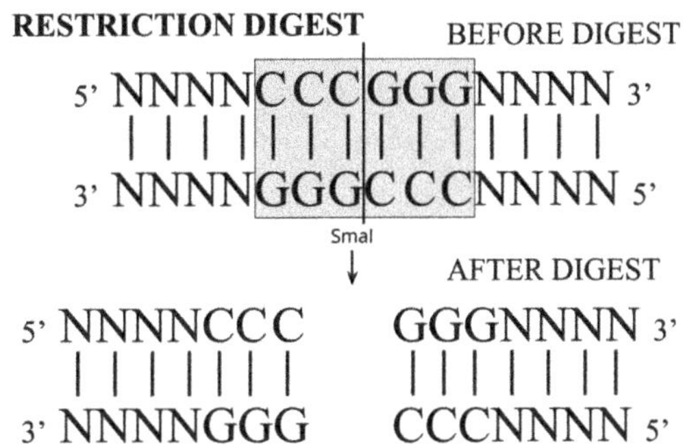

Fig. 2 Restriction enzyme digest of CCCGGG using SmaI producing two blunt ends. In general, DNA is represented as a permutation of the four nucleotides [adenine (A), thymine (T), cytosine (C), guanine (G)] and an ambiguous base (N)

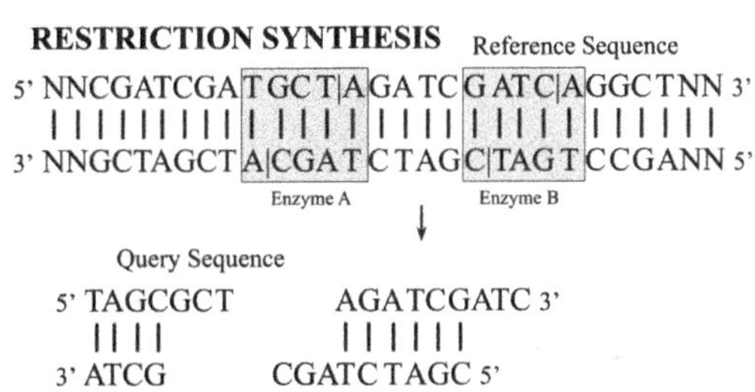

Fig. 3 Restriction synthesis. Reference sequence is flanked by Enzyme A and Enzyme B. This fragment is then ligated to the end of the query sequence

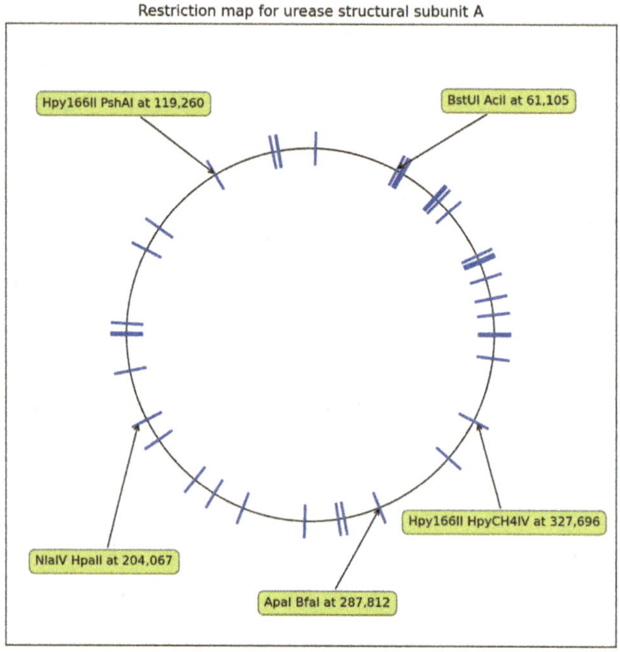

Fig. 4 Restriction map for the synthesis of Mycobacterium tuberculosis Erdman strain urease structural subunit A using restriction synthesis

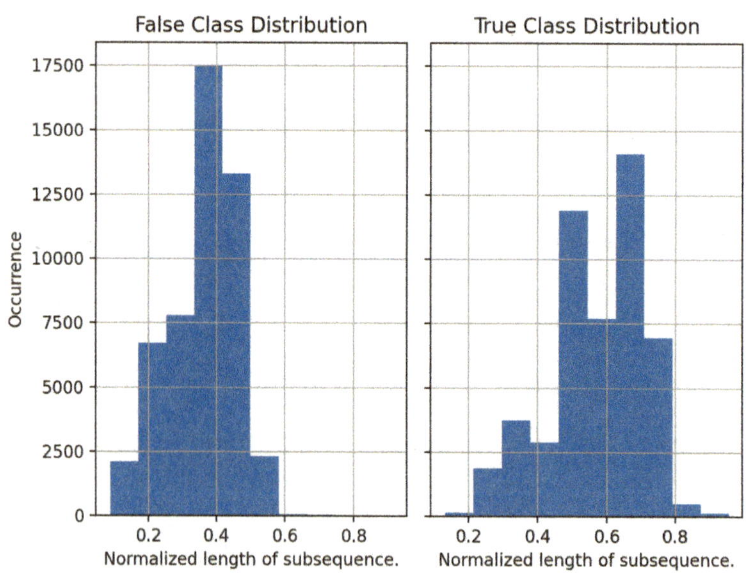

Fig. 5 Subsequence length feature distributions stratified by class label for subsequences

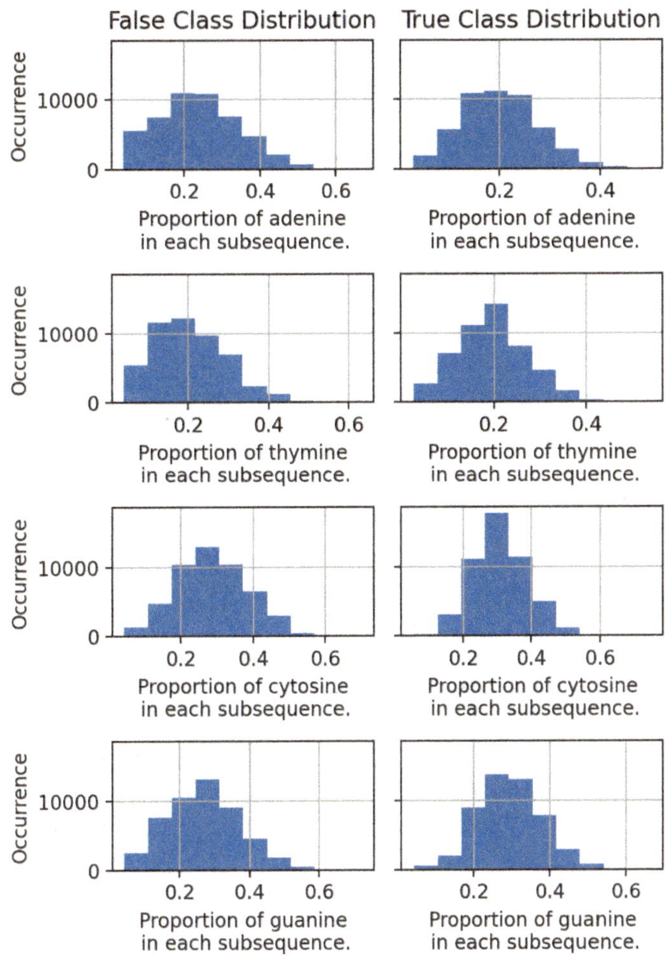

Fig. 6 Nucleotide proportion feature distributions stratified by class label for subsequences

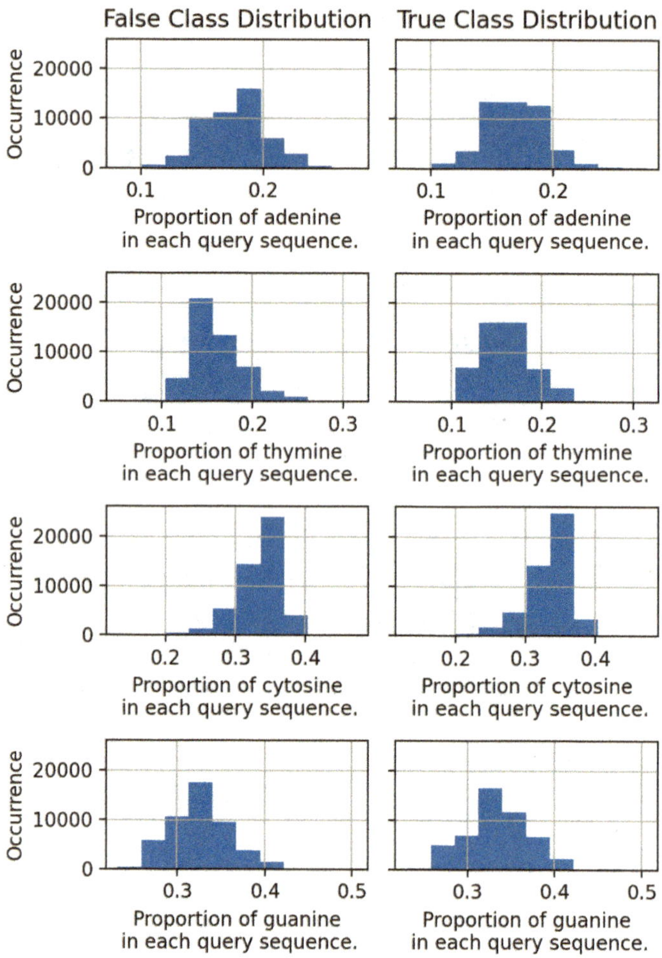

Fig. 7 Nucleotide proportion feature distributions stratified by class label for genes

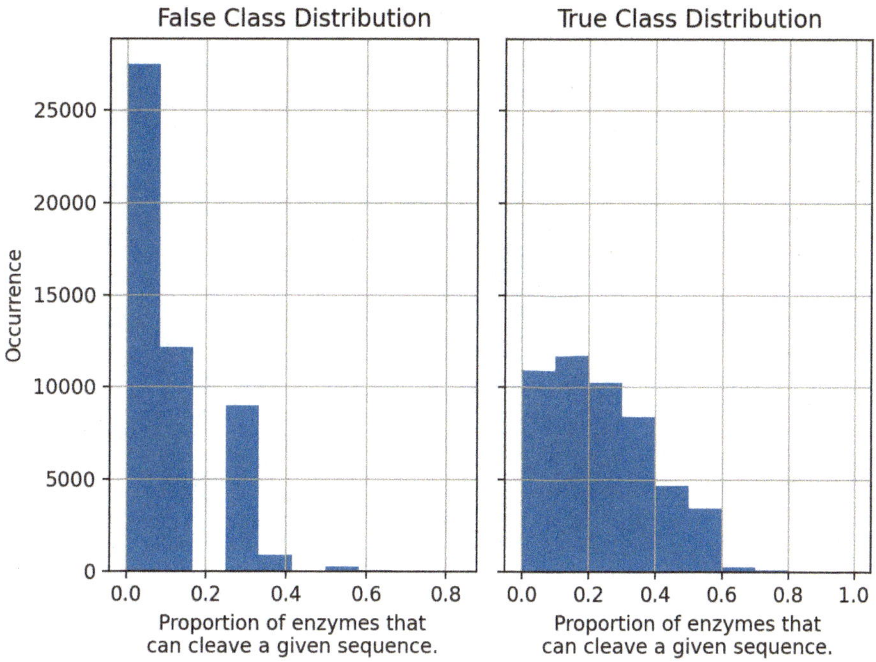

Fig. 8 Enzyme availability feature distributions stratified by class label for subsequences

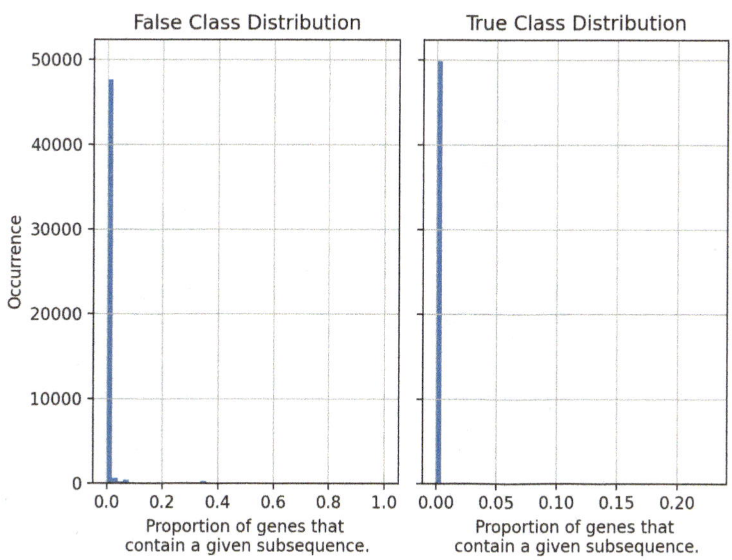

Fig. 9 Commonality feature distributions stratified by class label for subsequences

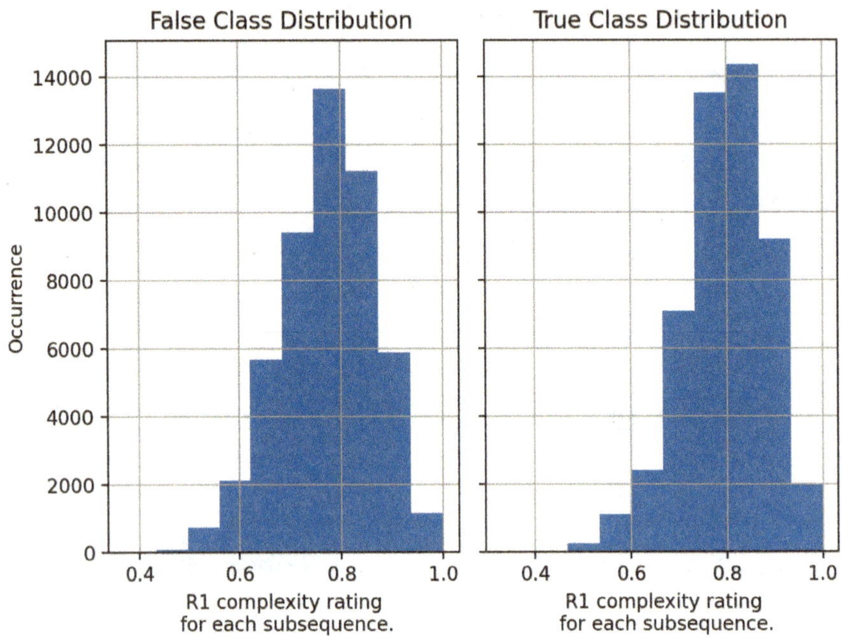

Fig. 10 R_1 feature distributions stratified by class label for subsequences

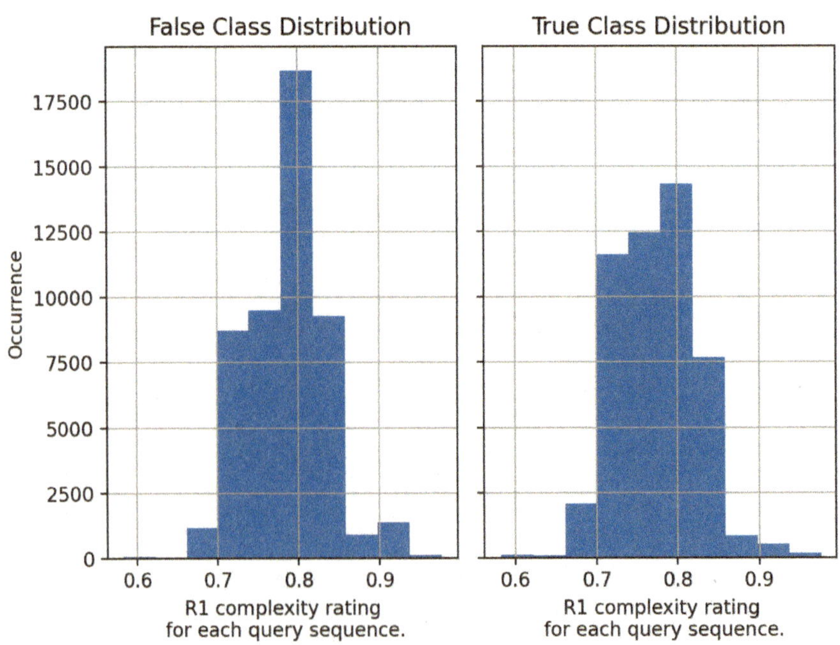

Fig. 11 R_2 feature distributions stratified by class label for subsequences

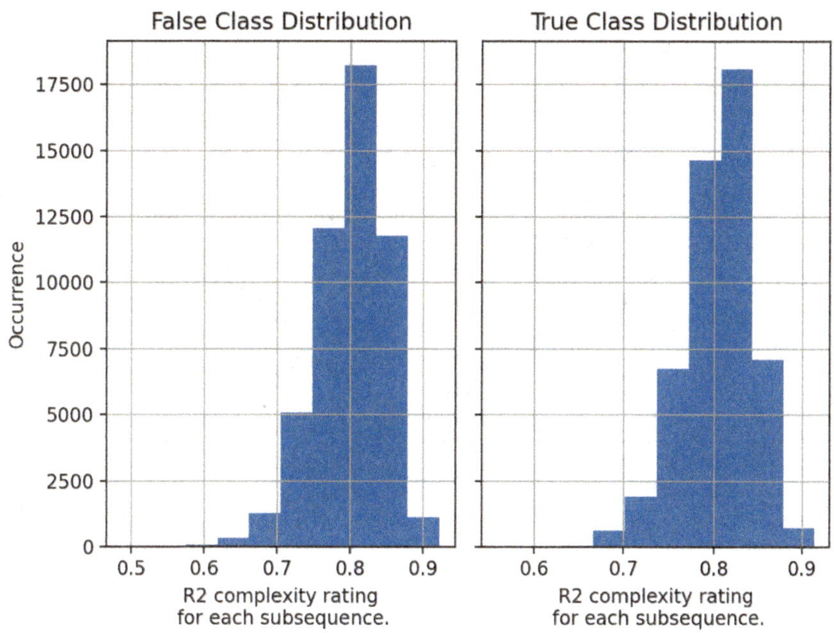

Fig. 12 R_1 feature distributions stratified by class label for genes

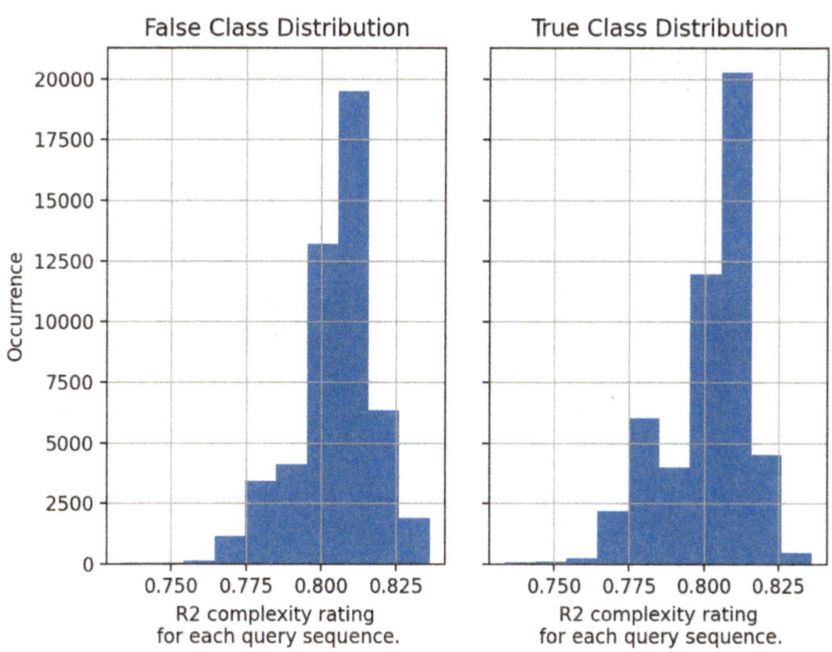

Fig. 13 R_2 feature distribution stratified by class label for genes

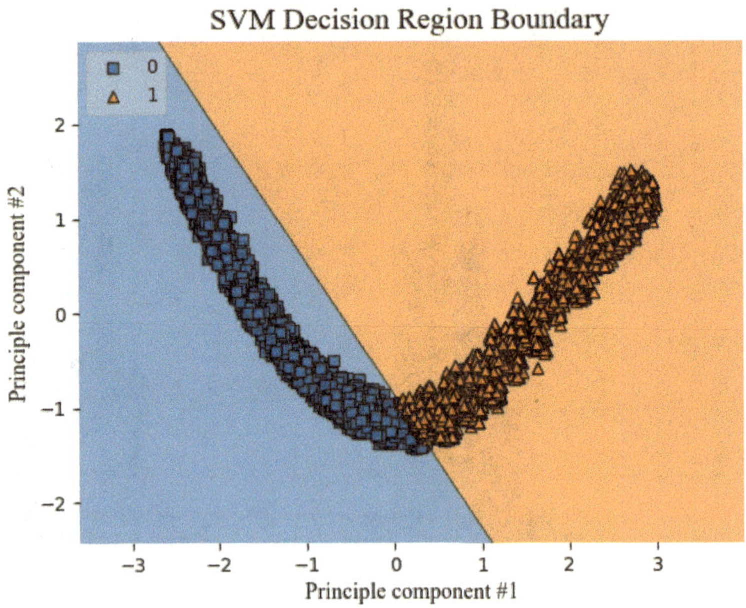

Fig. 14 Sample linear kernel 2 PCs SVM analysis

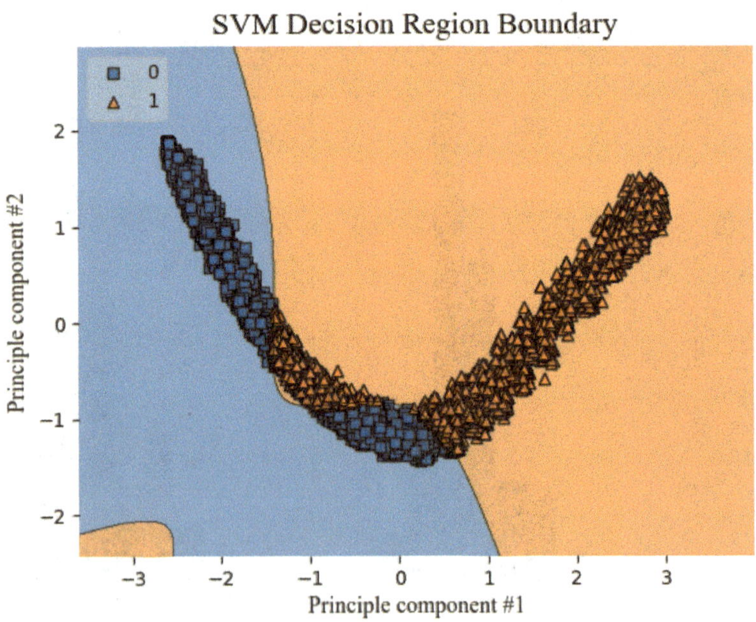

Fig. 15 Sample sigmoid kernel 2 PCs SVM analysis

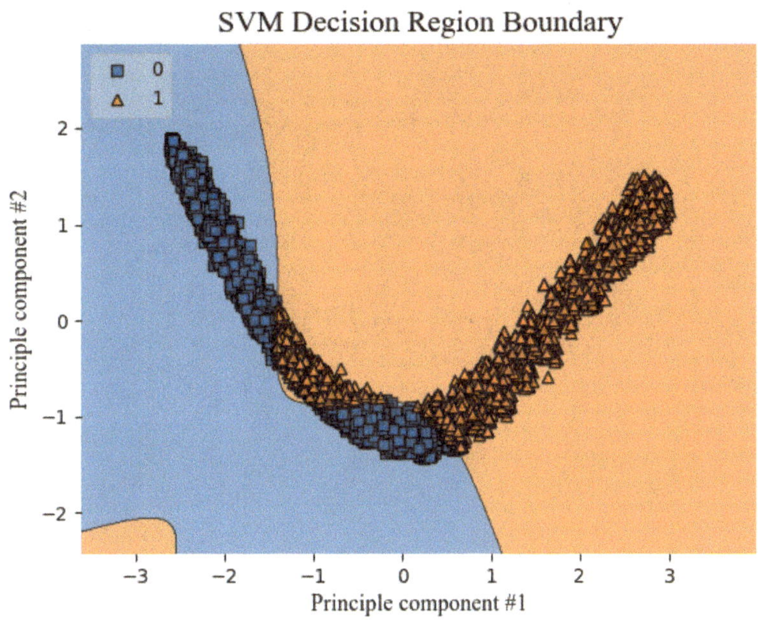

Fig. 16 Sample radial basis function (RBF) kernel 2 PCs SVM analysis

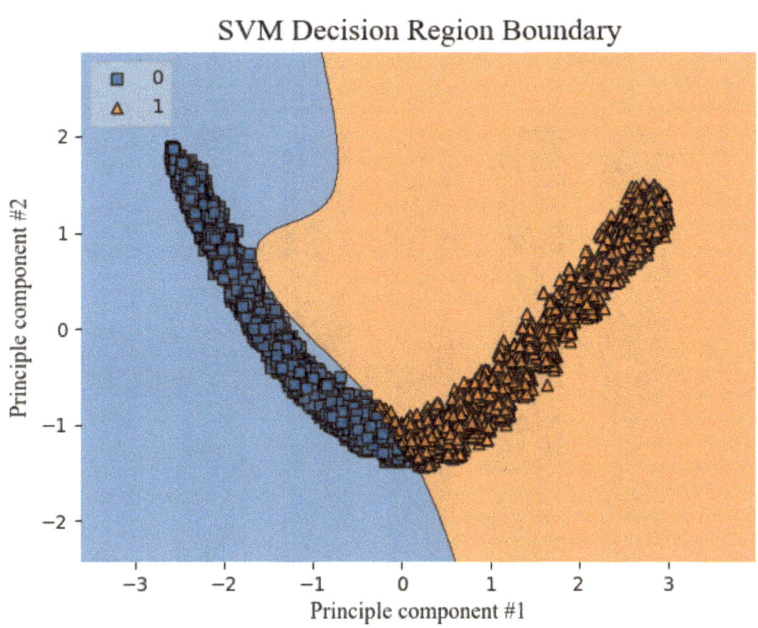

Fig. 17 Sample polymetric kernel 2 PCs SVM analysis

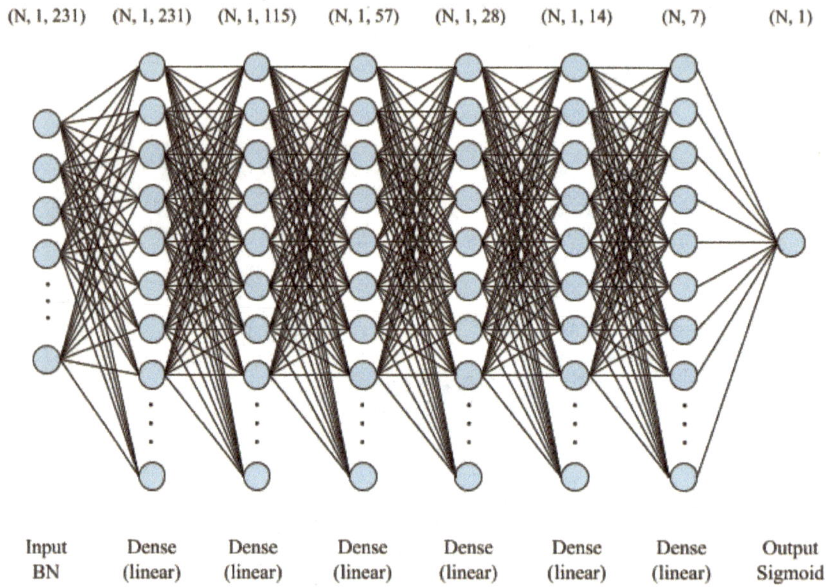

Fig. 18 Currently optimal ANN

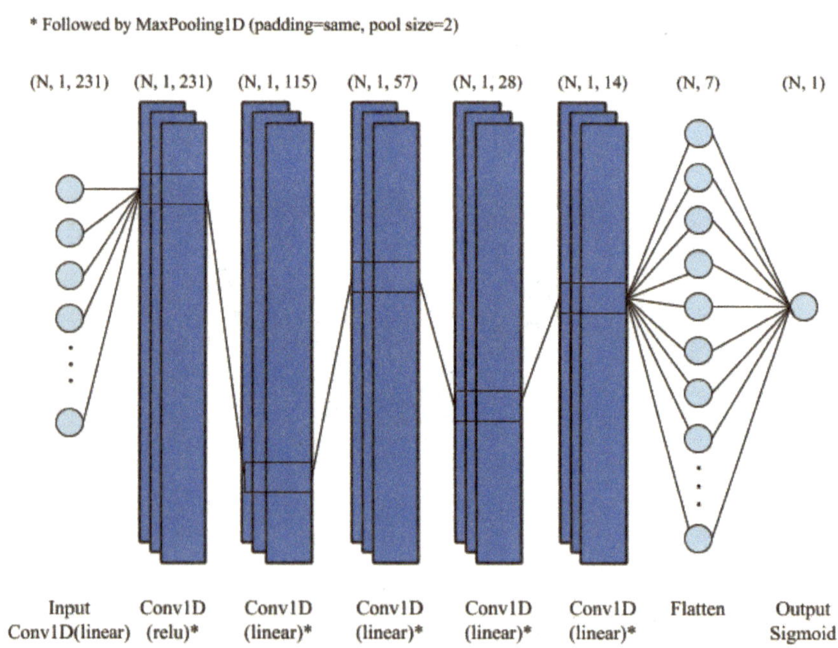

Fig. 19 Currently optimal CNN

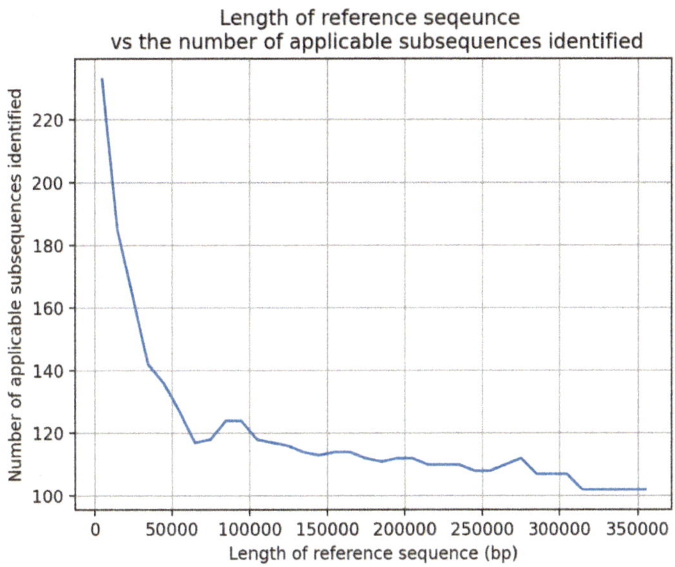

Fig. 20 Dependence of the number of applicable subsequences identified on the length of the randomized reference sequence for the restriction synthesis of Mycobacterium tuberculosis Erdman strain urease structural subunit

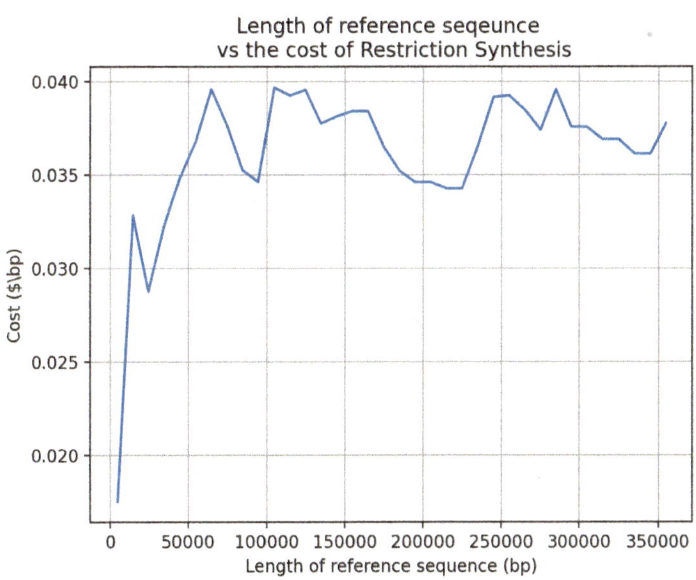

Fig. 21 Dependence of the cost of synthesis on the length of the randomized reference sequence for the restriction synthesis of Mycobacterium tuberculosis Erdman strain urease structural subunit

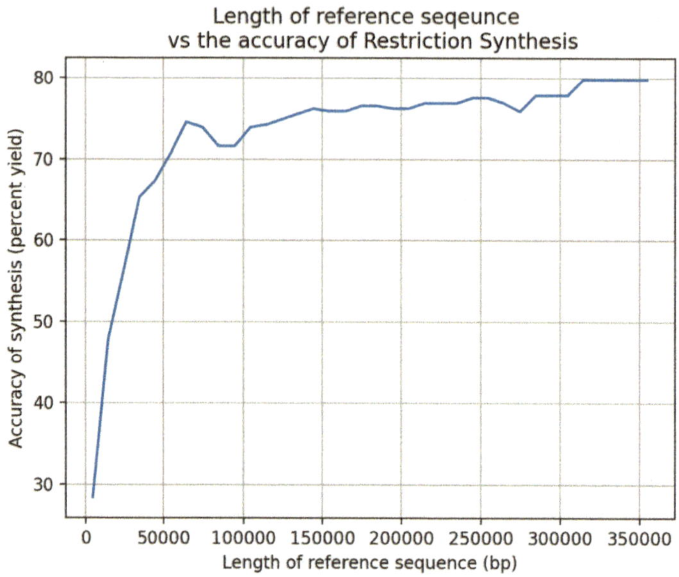

Fig. 22 Dependence of the accuracy of synthesis on the length of the randomized reference sequence for the restriction synthesis of Mycobacterium tuberculosis Erdman strain urease structural subunit

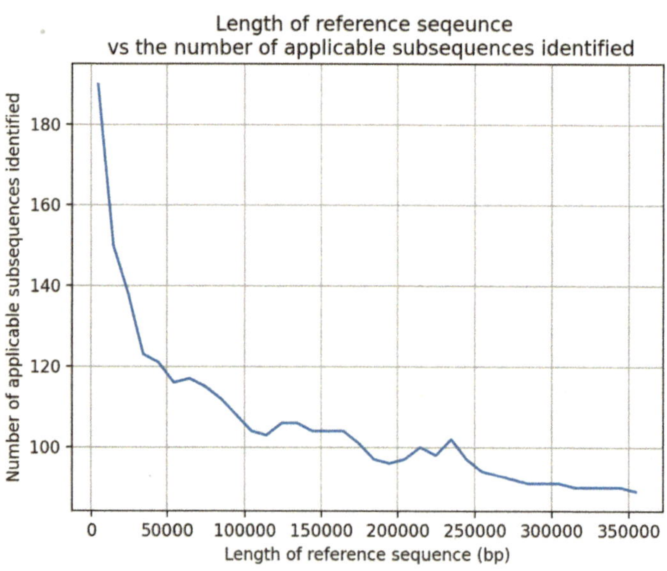

Fig. 23 Dependence of the number of applicable subsequences identified on the length of the generalized reference sequence for the restriction synthesis of Mycobacterium tuberculosis Erdman strain urease structural subunit

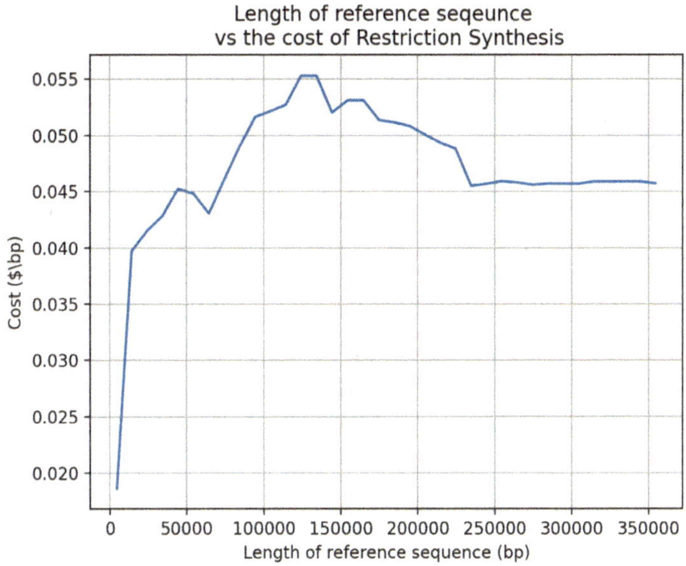

Fig. 24 Dependence of the cost of synthesis on the length of the generalized reference sequence for the restriction synthesis of Mycobacterium tuberculosis Erdman strain urease structural subunit

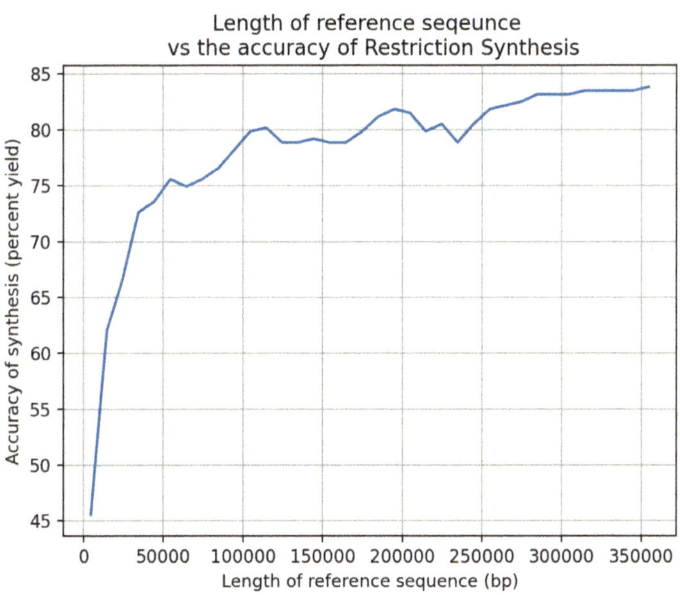

Fig. 25 Dependence of the accuracy of synthesis on the length of the generalized reference sequence for the restriction synthesis of Mycobacterium tuberculosis Erdman strain urease structural subunit

Table 1 General confusion matrix

	Actual true	Actual false
Predicted true	True positive	False positive
Predicted false	False negative	True negative

Table 2 Pairwise Pearson correlation test with non-nucleotide features

	LEN	P(A)	P(T)	P(C)	P(G)	R1	R2	C	gP(A)	gP(T)	gP(C)	gP(G)	gR1	gR2	EZY	Output
LEN	1	−0.124	0.03	0.039	0.057	0.244	0.049	−0.247	−0.158	0.003	−0.009	0.118	−0.108	−0.127	0.404	0.661
P(A)	−0.124	1	−0.205	−0.329	−0.487	0.213	0.083	0.093	0.217	−0.008	0.012	−0.158	0.147	0.104	−0.257	−0.208
P(T)	0.03	−0.205	1	−0.399	−0.301	0.364	0.15	0.018	0.023	0.111	−0.069	−0.044	0.093	0.093	−0.16	−0.055
P(C)	0.039	−0.329	−0.399	1	−0.274	−0.336	−0.163	−0.051	−0.046	−0.077	0.119	−0.007	−0.083	−0.096	0.223	0.134
P(G)	0.057	−0.487	−0.301	−0.274	1	−0.211	−0.059	−0.059	−0.189	−0.017	−0.064	0.2	−0.146	−0.094	0.181	0.125
R1	0.244	0.213	0.364	−0.336	−0.211	1	0.481	−0.028	0.032	0.073	−0.048	−0.038	0.074	0.079	−0.015	0.11
R2	0.049	0.083	0.15	−0.163	−0.059	0.481	1	−0.022	0.023	0.048	−0.022	−0.035	0.053	0.08	0.068	0.031
C	−0.247	0.093	0.018	−0.051	−0.059	−0.028	−0.022	1	0.125	−0.01	−0.041	−0.048	0.081	0.107	−0.094	−0.117
gP(A)	−0.158	0.217	0.023	−0.046	−0.189	0.032	0.023	0.125	1	0.006	−0.021	−0.702	0.7	0.364	−0.129	−0.162
gP(T)	0.003	−0.008	0.111	−0.077	−0.017	0.073	0.048	−0.01	0.006	1	−0.595	−0.272	0.704	0.501	−0.034	−0.01
gP(C)	−0.009	0.012	−0.069	0.119	−0.064	−0.048	−0.022	−0.041	−0.021	−0.595	1	−0.355	−0.405	−0.267	0.012	−0.018
gP(G)	0.118	−0.158	−0.044	−0.007	0.2	−0.038	−0.035	−0.048	−0.702	−0.272	−0.355	1	−0.701	−0.418	0.108	0.137
gR1	−0.108	0.147	0.093	−0.083	−0.146	0.074	0.053	0.081	0.7	0.704	−0.405	−0.701	1	0.631	−0.111	−0.12
gR2	−0.127	0.104	0.093	−0.096	−0.094	0.079	0.08	0.107	0.364	0.501	−0.267	−0.418	0.631	1	−0.064	−0.119
EZY	0.404	−0.257	−0.16	0.223	0.181	−0.015	0.068	−0.094	−0.129	−0.034	0.012	0.108	−0.111	−0.064	1	0.411
Output	0.661	−0.208	−0.055	0.134	0.125	0.11	0.031	−0.117	−0.162	−0.01	−0.018	0.137	−0.12	−0.119	0.411	1

Table 3 Highest correlated nucleotide features

Feature	Highest correlated feature	Correlation
Nuc1	Nuc4	0.114
Nuc2	Nuc1	0.066
Nuc3	Nuc6	0.047
Nuc4	Nuc1	0.114
Nuc5	Nuc8	0.049
Nuc6	Nuc9	0.064
Nuc7	Nuc10	0.109
Nuc8	Nuc9	0.138
Nuc9	Nuc10	0.197
Nuc10	Nuc11	0.241
Nuc11	Nuc12	0.351
Nuc12	Nuc15	0.405
Nuc13	Nuc14	0.433
Nuc14	Nuc15	0.439
Nuc15	Nuc16	0.506
Nuc16	Nuc17	0.549
Nuc17	Nuc18	0.59
Nuc18	Nuc19	0.602
Nuc19	Nuc18	0.602
Nuc20	Nuc21	0.639
Nuc21	Nuc20	0.639
Nuc22	Nuc21	0.635
Nuc23	Nuc24	0.682
Nuc24	Nuc25	0.695
Nuc25	Nuc26	0.726
Nuc26	Nuc27	0.733
Nuc27	Nuc28	0.779
Nuc28	Nuc27	0.779
Nuc29	Nuc28	0.725
Nuc30	Nuc29	0.702
Nuc31	Nuc29	0.561
Nuc32	Nuc31	0.51
Nuc33	Nuc32	0.439
Nuc34	Nuc35	0.509
Nuc35	Nuc36	0.563
Nuc36	Nuc37	0.656
Nuc37	Nuc38	0.723
Nuc38	Nuc37	0.723
Nuc39	Nuc40	0.638
Nuc40	Nuc41	0.886
Nuc41	Nuc40	0.886
Nuc42	Nuc41	0.757
Nuc43	Nuc42	0.755

Table 4 Lowest correlated nucleotide features

Feature	Lowest correlated feature	Correlation
Nuc1	Nuc3	−0.053
Nuc2	Nuc3	−0.018
Nuc3	Nuc28	−0.115
Nuc4	Nuc40	−0.038
Nuc5	Nuc22	−0.031
Nuc6	Nuc28	−0.053
Nuc7	Nuc30	−0.024
Nuc8	Nuc3	−0.012
Nuc9	Nuc36	−0.033
Nuc10	Nuc3	−0.03
Nuc11	Nuc3	−0.045
Nuc12	Nuc3	−0.027
Nuc13	Nuc3	−0.05
Nuc14	Nuc3	−0.065
Nuc15	Nuc3	−0.057
Nuc16	Nuc3	−0.068
Nuc17	Nuc3	−0.063
Nuc18	Nuc3	−0.087
Nuc19	Nuc3	−0.081
Nuc20	Nuc3	−0.064
Nuc21	Nuc3	−0.063
Nuc22	Nuc3	−0.07
Nuc23	Nuc3	−0.063
Nuc24	Nuc3	−0.079
Nuc25	Nuc3	−0.078
Nuc26	Nuc3	−0.094
Nuc27	Nuc3	−0.093
Nuc28	Nuc3	−0.115
Nuc29	Nuc3	−0.093
Nuc30	Nuc3	−0.101
Nuc31	Nuc3	−0.088
Nuc32	Nuc3	−0.059
Nuc33	Nuc3	−0.041
Nuc34	Nuc3	−0.016
Nuc35	Nuc4	−0.022
Nuc36	Nuc9	−0.033
Nuc37	Nuc9	−0.021
Nuc38	Nuc3	−0.024
Nuc39	Nuc4	−0.019
Nuc40	Nuc4	−0.038
Nuc41	Nuc4	−0.038
Nuc42	Nuc4	−0.033
Nuc43	Nuc4	−0.033

Table 5 Pairwise Pearson correlation with nucleotide features for sequences 10 base pairs and less

	Nuc1	Nuc2	Nuc3	Nuc4	Nuc5	Nuc6	Nuc7	Nuc8	Nuc9	Nuc10
Nuc1	1.000	0.187	−0.182	0.249	0.038	−0.030	0.148	0.135	0.207	0.199
Nuc2	0.187	1.000	−0.022	−0.059	0.117	0.136	0.163	0.127	0.138	0.133
Nuc3	−0.182	−0.022	1.000	−0.210	0.033	0.198	0.015	0.044	−0.036	−0.028
Nuc4	0.249	−0.059	−0.210	1.000	−0.158	−0.161	0.029	−0.021	0.059	0.046
Nuc5	0.038	0.117	0.033	−0.158	1.000	0.281	0.185	0.234	0.160	0.077
Nuc6	−0.030	0.136	0.198	−0.161	0.281	1.000	0.289	0.188	0.226	0.108
Nuc7	0.148	0.163	0.015	0.029	0.185	0.289	1.000	0.471	0.369	0.319
Nuc8	0.135	0.127	0.044	−0.021	0.234	0.188	0.471	1.000	0.472	0.261
Nuc9	0.207	0.138	−0.036	0.059	0.160	0.226	0.369	0.472	1.000	0.467
Nuc10	0.199	0.133	−0.028	0.046	0.077	0.108	0.319	0.261	0.467	1.000

Table 6 Support Vector Machine model results for Linear Kernel, Sigmoid Kernel, Radial Basis Function (RBF) Kernel, and Polymetric Kernel without Principal Component Analysis

	Accuracy (%)	Precision (%)	Recall (%)	F1-measure
Linear Kernel	87.97	83.07	92.10	87.35
Sigmoid Kernel	79.00	77.90	79.65	78.76
RBF	93.33	91.36	95.10	93.19
Polymetric Kernel	**94.09**	**92.80**	**95.25**	**94.01**

Table 7 Support Vector Machine model results for Linear Kernel, Sigmoid Kernel, Radial Basis Function (RBF) Kernel, and Polymetric Kernel with Principal Component Analysis using two and three Principal Components (PCs). The maximum value for each metric is highlighted in bold

	Accuracy (%)	Precision (%)	Recall (%)	F1-measure
Linear Kernel (2 PC)	85.99	78.48	92.35	84.85
Sigmoid Kernel (2 PC)	76.46	76.38	76.51	76.44
RBF (2 PC)	87.63	81.40	92.99	86.81
Polymetric Kernel (2 PC)	86.20	**82.79**	88.85	85.71
Linear Kernel (3 PC)	86.09	78.54	92.51	84.95
Sigmoid Kernel (3 PC)	78.30	78.25	78.33	78.29
RBF (3 PC)	**87.76**	81.40	**93.27**	**86.93**
Polymetric Kernel (3 PC)	87.19	82.05	91.44	86.49

Table 8 Random Forest results for $n = 10, 15, \ldots 55, 65$ with 10-fold cross validation results. The maximum value for each metric is highlighted in bold

	Accuracy (%)	Precision (%)	Recall (%)	F1-measure
Random Forest (n=10)	94.96	93.00	96.80	94.86
Random Forest (n=15)	95.19	93.91	96.37	95.13
Random Forest (n=20)	95.31	93.65	96.87	95.23
Random Forest (n=25)	95.36	94.01	96.62	95.30
Random Forest (n=30)	95.39	93.74	96.93	95.31
Random Forest (n=35)	95.39	94.00	96.68	95.33
Random Forest (n=40)	95.44	93.93	96.86	95.37
Random Forest (n=45)	**95.53**	**94.12**	96.86	**95.47**
Random Forest (n=50)	95.51	93.92	**97.01**	95.44

Table 9 K-Nearest Neighbor results for $k = 3, 5, 7, 9, 11$ with 10-fold cross validation results. The maximum value for each metric is highlighted in bold

	Accuracy (%)	Precision (%)	Recall (%)	F1-measure
KNN (k=1)	93.00	**93.21**	**92.81**	93.01
KNN (k=3)	**93.15**	93.14	93.16	**93.15**
KNN (k=5)	92.84	92.49	93.15	92.82
KNN (k=7)	92.65	92.04	93.18	92.61
KNN (k=9)	92.41	91.58	93.13	92.35
KNN (k=11)	92.23	91.16	93.16	92.15

Table 10 Artificial Neural Network results using only nucleotide features and all available features with 10-fold cross validation results. The maximum value for each metric is highlighted in bold

	Accuracy (%)	Precision (%)	Recall (%)	F1-measure
ANN (all features)	**95.20**	**95.41**	95.01	**95.21**
ANN (nucleotide features)	95.08	94.92	**95.24**	95.07

Table 11 Convolutional Neural Network results using only nucleotide features and all available features with 10-fold cross validation results. The maximum value for each metric is highlighted in bold

	Accuracy (%)	Precision (%)	Recall (%)	F1-measure
CNN (all features)	94.80	94.25	**95.32**	94.77
CNN (nucleotide features)	**94.90**	**94.77**	95.02	**94.89**

Table 12 Best performing machine learning models with 10-fold cross validation

	Accuracy (%)	Precision (%)	Recall (%)	F1-measure
SVM (RBF 3 PC)	87.76	81.40	93.27	86.93
Random Forest (n=45)	**95.53**	94.12	**96.86**	**95.47**
Naive Bayes	78.87	58.84	98.16	73.58
KNN (k=3)	93.15	93.14	93.16	93.15
ANN (all features)	95.20	**95.41**	95.01	95.21
CNN (nucleotide features)	94.90	94.77	95.02	94.89

References

1. National Center for Biotechnology Information. (2020). Gene [Internet]. Bethesda (MD): National Library of Medicine (US), National Center for Biotechnology Information, 2020.
2. Watson, J. D., & Crick, F. H. C. (1953). Genetical implications of the structure of deoxyribonucleic acid. *Nature, 171*, 964–967.
3. Tatum, W., & Hausman, R. E. (2000). *The Cell: A Molecular Approach, Sixth Edition.* Sunderland, MA: Sinauer Associates, Inc.
4. Reichard, P. (1988). Interactions between deoxyribonucleotide and dna synthesis. *Annual Review of Biochemistry, 57*(1), 349–374.
5. Hughes, R. A., & Ellington, A. D. (2017). Synthetic DNA synthesis and assembly: Putting the synthetic in synthetic biology. *Cold Spring Harbor Perspectives in Biology, 9*(1), a023812.
6. Caruthers, M. H. (1985). Gene synthesis machines: DNA chemistry and its uses. *Science, 230*(4723), 281–285.
7. Jensen, M. A., & Davis, R. W. (2018). Template-independent enzymatic oligonucleotide synthesis (TiEOS): its history, prospects, and challenges. *ACS Publications*, 1821–1832.
8. National Human Genome Research Institute. (2020). The Human Genome Project, 2020.
9. Broad Institute. (2020). CRISPR Timeline, 2020.
10. Nicholas, T., Siying, M., & Jingdong, T. (2013). Chapter 1 - New tools for cost-effective DNA synthesis. In H. Zhao, (Ed.), *Synthetic Biology* (pp. 3–21).
11. Dias, N., & Stein, C. A. (2002). Antisense oligonucleotides: Basic concepts and mechanisms. *Molecular Cancer Therapeutics*, 347–355.
12. Biobasic. (2021) Pricing | Gene Synthesis.
13. Bigger, C. H., Murray, K., & Murray, N. E. (1973). Recognition sequence of a restriction enzyme. *Nature New Biology, 244*(131), 7–10.
14. New England Biolabs. (2021). Restriction Isoschizomers, 2021.
15. New England Biolabs. (2021). Blunting, 2021.
16. Shetty, R. P., Endy, D., & Knight, T. F. (2008). Engineering biobrick vectors from biobrick parts. *Journal of Biological Engineering, 2*(1), 5.
17. Anderson, J.C., et al. (2010). Bglbricks: A flexible standard for biological part assembly. *Journal of Biological Engineering, 4*(1), 1.
18. New England Biolabs. (2020) Restriction Endonucleases, 2020.
19. Liu, Q., Dang, H.-J., Wu, Y.-H., Li, M., Chen, Y.-H., Niu, X.-L., Li, K.-M., & Luo, L.-J. (2018). pXST, a novel vector for TA cloning and blunt-end cloning. *BMC Biotechnology, 18*(1), 1–7. BioMed Central.
20. Cadwell, R. C., & Joyce, G. F. (1992). *Randomization of genes by PCR mutagenesis*. La Jolla, CA: Departments of Chemistry and Molecular Biology, The Scripps Research Institute, The Scripps Research Institute.
21. McCullum, O. E., Williams, B. A. R., Zhang, J., & Chaput, J. C. (2018). *Random mutagenesis by error-prone PCR*. Irvine: University of California.

22. Bosco, G. L., & Gangi, M. A. D. (2017). Deep learning architectures for DNA sequence classification. *Fuzzy Logic and Soft Computing Applications*, 162–171.
23. Nguyen, N., et al. (2016). DNA sequence classification by convolutional neural network. *Journal Biomedical Science and Engineering*, 280–286.
24. Rizzo, R., Fiannaca, A., Massimo, L. R., & Urso, A. (2016). A deep learning approach to DNA sequence classification. *Computational Intelligence Methods for Bioinformatics and Biostatistics*, 129–140.
25. Phan, D., et al. (2017). Combined use of k-Mer numerical features and position-specific categorical features in fixed-length DNA sequence classification. *Journal of Biomedical Science and Engineering, 10*(8), 390–401.
26. GensSript. (2021). GenBrick gene synthesis service for synthetic biology. *www.genscript.com*.
27. Suykens, J. A. K., & Vandewalle, J. (1999). Least squares support vector machine classifiers. *Neural Processing Letters, 9*(3), 293–300.
28. Noble, W. S. (2006). What is a support vector machine? *Nature Biotechnology, 24*(12), 1565–1567.
29. Yao, B., Hu, P., Zhang, M., & Jin, M. (2014). A support vector machine with the tabu search algorithm for freeway incident detection. *International Journal of Applied Mathematics and Computer Science, 24*(2), 397–404.
30. Boyle, B. H. (2011). *Support vector machines: data analysis, machine learning and applications*. Nova Science Publishers, Inc.
31. Lever, J., Krzywinski, M., & Altman, N. (2017). Principal component analysis. *Nature Methods, 14*(7), 641–642.
32. Pal, M. (2005). Random forest classifier for remote sensing classification. *International Journal of Remote Sensing, 26*(1), 217–222.
33. Liaw, A., Wiener, M., et al. (2002). Classification and regression by randomforest. *R News, 2*(3), 18–22.
34. Breiman, L., & Cutler, A. (2020). *Random forests - Classification description*. Berkeley University.
35. Cutler, A., & Stevens, J. R. (2006). Random forests for microarrays. In *DNA microarrays, Part B: Databases and statistics*, volume 411 of *Methods in enzymology* (pp. 422–432).
36. Devetyarov, D., & Nouretdinov, I. (2010). Prediction with confidence based on a random forest classifier. In *IFIP international conference on artificial intelligence applications and innovations* (pp. 37–44). Springer.
37. Rish, I., et al. (2001). An empirical study of the naive Bayes classifier. In *IJCAI 2001 workshop on empirical methods in artificial intelligence* (pp. 41–46).
38. Murphy, K., et al. (2006). Naive bayes classifiers. *University of British Columbia, 18*, 60.
39. Peterson, L. E. (2009). K-nearest neighbor. *Scholarpedia, 4*, 1883.
40. Zell, A. (2003). *Simulation Neuronaler Netze (Simulation with neuronal networks)*, chapter 5.2. Wissenschaftsverlag: Oldenbourg.
41. Abbod, M. F., Catto, J. W. F., Linkens, D. A., & Hamdy, F. C. (2007). Application of artificial intelligence to the management of urological cancer. *The Journal of Urology, 178*, 1150–1156. Elsevier.
42. Alparslan, Y., Moyer, E. J., Isozaki, I. M., Schwartz, D., Dunlop, A., Dave, S., & Kim, E. (2021). Towards searching efficient and accurate neural network architectures in binary classification problems. Preprint. arXiv:2101.06511.
43. Alparslan, Y., Moyer, E. J., & Kim, E. (2021). Evaluating online and offline accuracy traversal algorithms for k-complete neural network architectures. Preprint. arXiv:2101.06518.
44. Goodfellow, I., Bengio, Y., & Courville, A. (2016). *Deep learning*. MIT Press.
45. Schmidhuber, J. (2015). Deep learning in neural networks: An overview. *Neural Networks, 61*, 85–117.
46. LeCun, Y., Bengio, Y., & Hinton, G. (2015). Deep learning. *Nature, 521*, 436–444.
47. Bengio, Y., Goodfellow, I., & Courville, A. (2017). *Deep learning*, volume 1. MA, USA: MIT Press.

48. Ciregan, D., Meier, U., & Schmidhuber, J. (2012). Multi-column deep neural networks for image classification. In *2012 IEEE conference on computer vision and pattern recognition* (pp. 3642–3649).
49. Baccouche, M., Mamalet, F., Wolf, C., Garcia, C., & Baskurt, A. (2011). Sequential deep learning for human action recognition. In *International workshop on human behavior understanding* (pp. 29–39). Springer.
50. Virmani, S., & Gite, S. (2017). Performance of convolutional neural network and recurrent neural network for anticipation of driver's conduct. In *2017 8th international conference on computing, communication and networking technologies (ICCCNT)* (pp. 1–8). IEEE.
51. Bai, S., Kolter, J. Z., & Koltun, V. (2018). An empirical evaluation of generic convolutional and recurrent networks for sequence modeling. Preprint. arXiv:1803.01271.
52. Moyer, E. J., & Das, A. (2021). Motif identification using CNN-based pairwise subsequence alignment score prediction. Preprint. arXiv:2101.08385.
53. Buhmann, M. D. (2021). Radial basis functions. *Acta Numerica, 9*, 1–38. Cambridge University Press.
54. Santurkar, S., Tsipras, D., Ilyas, A., & Madry, A. (2017). How does batch normalization help optimization? *Advances in Neural Information Processing Systems*, 2483–2493.
55. Team Keras. (2021). Adam Optimizer. https://keras.io/api/optimizers/adam/.
56. Valueva, M. V., Nagornov, N. N., Lyakhov, P. A., Valuev, G. V., & Chervyakov, N. I. (2020). Application of the residue number system to reduce hardware costs of the convolutional neural network implementation. *Mathematics and Computers in Simulation, 177*, 232–243. Elsevier.
57. Tsantekidis, A., Passalis, N., Tefas, A., Kanniainen, J., Gabbouj, M., & Iosifidis, A. (2018). AForecasting stock prices from the limit order book using convolutional neural networks. In *2017 IEEE 19th conference on business informatics (CBI)* (vol. 1, pp. 7–12). IEEE.
58. Kodumal, S. J., Patel, K. G., Reid, R., Menzella, H. G., Welch, M., & Santi, D. V. (2004). Total synthesis of long DNA sequences: synthesis of a contiguous 32-kb polyketide synthase gene cluster. *Proceedings of the National Academy of Sciences, 101*, 15573–15578.
59. Brown, T., Brown, T. Jr., Brown, B., & Brown, A. (2018). Solid-phase oligonucleotide synthesis. *Atdbio.Com*.
60. Laikhter, A., & Linse, K. D. (2014). The chemical synthesis of oligonucleotides. *biosyn.com*.
61. Blackburn, M., Gait, M. J., Loakes, D., & Williams, D. M. (2007). Nucleic acids in chemistry and biology: Edition 3. *Vilnius University*.

Human Detection and Biometric Authentication with Ambient Sensors

Jack Andrews and Jia Li

Abbreviations

AD	Alzheimer's disease
AI	Artificial intelligence
ANN	Artificial neural network
CM-PIR	Chest motion passive infrared sensor
CNN	Convolutional neural network
COTS	Commercial-off-the-shelf
CSI	Channel state information
DL	Deep learning
DWT	Discrete wavelet transform
ECG	Electrocardiogram
FFT	Fast Fourier transform
FN	False negative
FOV	Field of view
FP	False positive
GPR	Gaussian process regression
HAR	Human activity recognition
IDE	Integrated development environment
IOT	Internet of things
LSTM	Long-short term memory
MI-PIR	Motion induced passive infrared sensor
ML	Machine learning
PCA	Principal component analysis

J. Andrews (✉) · J. Li
Department of Electrical and Computer Engineering, Oakland University, Rochester, MI, USA
e-mail: jackandrews@oakland.edu

I. Obeid et al. (eds.), *Biomedical Sensing and Analysis*,
https://doi.org/10.1007/978-3-030-99383-2_2

PD	Parkinson's disease
PIR	Passive infrared
RELU	Rectified linear unit
RF	Radio frequency
RFID	Radio frequency identification
RNN	Recurrent neural network
RSSI	Received signal strength indicator
SGD	Stochastic gradient descent
TN	True negative
TP	True positive

1 Introduction

The geriatric population continues to increase and place a large burden on the healthcare systems worldwide. In 2019, there were 703 million people aged 65 or older across the globe. By 2050, this number is expected to double to an expected 1.5 billion people [1]. This increase in population is due to changes in lifestyle, the aging Baby Boomer generation, and increasing medical advancements, among other causes [2]. By 2030, the entire Baby Boomer generation will be older than 65 years of age and at that point, for the first time in the history of the United States, elderly people will outnumber the child generation. As evidence, by 2034, there will be 77 million people 65 years and older compared to 76.5 million people under the age of 18 [3]. The population older than 65 years of age currently accounts for 35% of all medical spending in the United States, indicating how the change in the population demographics may further impact the medical spending across the United States federal funding and health systems [4]. Many of these individuals are admitted to the hospital system for assistive care, as many normal activities can no longer be performed alone due to potential falls and memory loss [2].

Neurodegenerative diseases include dementia, Alzheimer's disease (AD), Parkinson's disease (PD), among various others. Largely due to these diseases, geriatric populations require additional assistance from a caregiver or admission to a long-term care facility site. Neurodegenerative diseases are complex in their pathophysiology, as some diseases cause memory and cognitive impairments, where others effect speaking and gait ability [5]. Due to this progressive degeneration in motor stability and memory, many of those that suffer from neurodegenerative diseases are prone to falls and memory loss effects [6]. For an insight into the number of people who suffer from neurodegenerative diseases in the United States, in 2015, five million suffered from AD and one million suffered from PD [7]. Aging individuals, especially those suffering from neurodegenerative diseases, generally require assistive care for safe long-term living.

For safe and secure living in these presented populations, a caregiver or hospital stay is often required, which causes financial burdens on both the families and the healthcare system. With an increasing number of people in these categories, the financial burdens will continuously increase. There exists a need for remote monitoring systems to aid caregivers and hospital systems to allow for greater independence and alleviate the burden of these populations on the healthcare system. There exist many proposed systems for remote monitoring of geriatric populations in at-home environments in current research and in industry. Proposed solutions often utilize ambient sensors and artificial intelligence (AI) algorithms for accurate monitoring of the environment. Many of these systems rely on video-based modalities which raise privacy concerns for the monitored person. In addition, many systems rely on expensive hardware or difficult set-up with multiple sensors deployed throughout the home. Some systems utilize active sensors that raise some energy and health concerns as well. An accurate, non-intrusive, passive, inexpensive, and ubiquitous monitoring system for an at-home environment could solve these aforementioned shortcomings.

The utilization of ambient sensors and AI extends from the need of human monitoring applications to security and biometric authentication applications. With the advent of the internet of things (IoT), there exists a need for an enhanced sense of security of personal data. IoT specifically refers to the interconnection of the devices used in everyday life including kitchen items, beds, phones, cars, and televisions [8]. IoT is expected to continue to increase as well, as in 2030 an estimated 500 billion devices will be connected to the Internet [9]. The security of the ever-increasing number of connected devices in our daily life remains a challenge, as potential adversaries can take advantage of personal data, as well gain entrance to medications or personal belongings [8]. To protect the security of IoT devices, passwords are often utilized, but they can often be forgotten or stolen. Facial recognition and fingerprinting technologies have become popular and have reached consumer IoT devices as alternatives to written passwords, as seen in common Apple products. However, these too can be unreliable and forged [10, 11]. For instance, once a fingerprint is stolen or retrieved from a touched surface, the fingerprint will forever be compromised [12]. A whole sector of security using biological characteristics is referred to as biometrics and can be used for authentication and identification of individuals for increased security of IoT devices. Where passwords can be forgotten or stolen, biometrics are unique to one individual person and are more difficult to replicate [8].

Biometric authentication refers to the use of a unique biological quality to confirm one person's identity against all other potential adversaries, while biometric identification classifies every individual in the dataset as unique. Common biometrics include previously mentioned fingerprints and facial recognition with additional unique characteristics including iris, gait, and voice. These biometrics are used to enhance the security of IoT devices, in comparison to written passwords or PIN numbers. Biometrics can be captured via non-contact sensors, such as in the case of cameras for facial recognition. Cameras, however, raise privacy concerns to the end-user. Therefore, a non-contact sensor for biometric authentication that alleviates the privacy intrusion to the end-user is seen as a superior modality for this purpose. With deep learning (DL), the collected biometrics from a non-contact sensor can be learned to differentiate a verified user against all other potential adversaries. To summarize, there exists a need for a secure, accurate, non-contact, and non-intrusive biometric authentication system to further enhance the security of IoT devices. Heart-related biometrics are growing in popularity, have shown promise as reliable for biometric authentication and identification systems, and could fill these mentioned shortcomings.

Various ambient sensors for non-contact sensing have been proposed for these applications including cameras, thermal sensors, depth sensors, and passive infrared (PIR) sensors. With the need for non-contact human monitoring and biometric authentication systems in mind, PIR sensors are inexpensive, commercial-off-the-shelf (COTS) components that are often utilized in monitoring and security applications. PIR sensors work by identifying the change in infrared radiation across its field of view (FoV) which is detected by the internal pyroelectric elements with alternating polarity. With everything above absolute zero temperature emitting some level of infrared radiation, theoretically any object in motion across a PIR sensor will be detected. As a result, human subjects in motion across a traditional PIR sensor will be detected. The major known drawback to PIR sensors, however, is the lack of reliable and accurate detection of stationary human subjects. For accurate use in human monitoring and biometric authentication situations, the inability to detect stationary human occupants will first have to be addressed.

To combat these mentioned drawbacks of human detection and biometric authentication systems, ambient sensors and AI have been proposed. Likewise, ambient signals have also garnished interest for non-contact monitoring including the likes of radio frequency (RF) and WiFi channel state information (CSI) for this purpose. DL algorithms including artificial neural networks (ANN), recurrent neural networks (RNN), and convolutional neural networks (CNN) have been utilized for learning of the sensor data for human detection and biometric authentication purposes. In our work, we propose using a PIR sensor as the ambient sensor with various statistical learning algorithms for human detection and biometric authentication classifications.

To address human detection and biometric authentication classifications via a single PIR sensor modality, we introduce and propose two novel systems in this work ...

1. Motion induced PIR sensor (MI-PIR)
2. Chest motion PIR sensor (CM-PIR)

Both systems are proposed to address the noted major known drawback of PIR sensors, which is the inability to reliably detect stationary human subjects [13, 14]. For MI-PIR, we extend the capabilities of this system from occupancy count estimation, relative location classification, and human target differentiation in one environment to precise indoor localization and human activity recognition (HAR) in two different ambient environments. For CM-PIR, we reintroduce the initial results of the biometric authentication system based on the chest motion data collected from 16 subjects at nine different home environments [14]. Human monitoring and biometric authentication via non-contact sensors and AI overall proves to have direct applications in medicine and healthcare as identified in assistive care living and security of private medical data from IoT devices. Accurate non-contact sensing systems will allow for long-term living in the elderly populations and more secure IoT devices, respectively.

2 Related Work

For accurate comparison of the two novel systems proposed in this work, many related systems will be introduced. For stationary human presence detection using PIR sensors, various solutions have been introduced, primarily those that rely on an optical shutter for accurate detection. Various additional ambient sensor modalities have been proposed for human monitoring and biometric authentication classifications that will also be highlighted in this section.

2.1 PIR Sensors

PIR sensors function by detecting the change in infrared radiation across its FoV. For binary PIR sensors, the change in infrared radiation will result in a "1" for a detected human subject and a "0" for no human subject detected. With infrared radiation being the resultant of temperatures greater than absolute zero temperature, other objects could potentially trigger a binary PIR sensor. For example, animals walking across the FoV of the PIR sensor, as well as a potential ball, car, or other object, could theoretically cause a false positive for a binary PIR sensor. When human bodies radiate infrared radiation from their body, there is a significant energy loss. The infrared radiation lost from a human body can be modeled by Eq. (1) below, which relates the energy loss from a blackbody (T) with its surroundings (T_S). In Eq. (1), the total power radiated from the human body (W_{tot}) is represented by this energy loss ($T^4 - {T_s}^4$) multiplied by the total surface area of the human in question (S) and the Stefan-Boltzmann constant (σ_{SB}) [15]. Eq. (1) proves the ambient environmental dependence on the infrared radiation of a human subject.

$$W_{tot} = S\sigma_{SB}\left(T^4 - T_s^4\right) \tag{1}$$

Analog PIR sensors output the voltage readings of the detected infrared radiation from a PIR sensor instead of the binary output, where an object in motion across the FoV will trigger a sinusoidal swing for the positive and negative terminals of the pyroelectric elements indicating human presence. For a typical human in motion, this will cause a swing to the maximum voltage and back to the minimum voltage; however, this sinusoidal swing is dependent on the mentioned ambient environment, and the motion and distance of the human subject. As a result, DL was proposed as a solution to learn from the varying outputs of the analog PIR sensor for various classifications including differentiating ambient environments, occupancy counts, human locations, and human subjects.

The FoV of a PIR sensor is generally expanded with the addition of a Fresnel lens. The Fresnel lens works to distribute the FoV of a PIR sensor into many evenly spaced fan-shaped zones with alternating polarities [16]. The Fresnel lens also works to expand the FoV of the PIR sensor by focusing the thermal image on

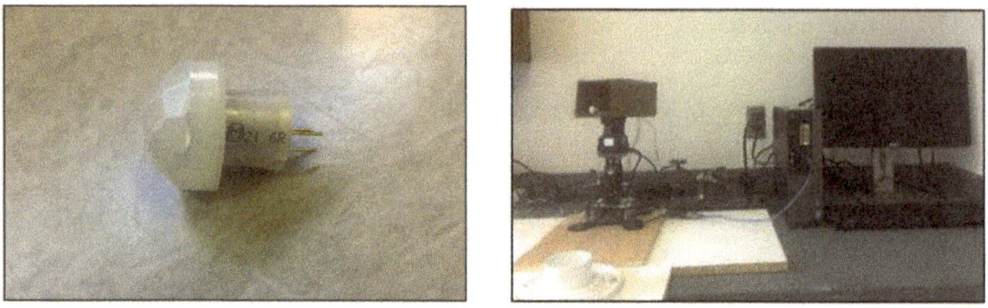

(a) (b)

Fig. 1 Novel MI-PIR system including the (**a**) the Panasonic AMN24112 and (**b**) the full design

the internal elements, which converts the thermal energy of the image into heat. Varying PIR sensors use different Fresnel lens and thus, there exist different FoV ranges for each PIR sensor [17]. In our work, we utilize the Panasonic AMN 24112 PIR sensor with analog output as identified in Fig. 1(a). The Fresnel lens on the Panasonic AMN 24112 PIR sensor expands the FoV to a recorded horizontal 93° and vertical 110°.

As stated, PIR sensors rely on a change in infrared radiation for accurate detection of a human subject. Due to this, stationary human subjects often go undetected and result in a major drawback to the deployment of PIR sensors in monitoring and security applications. To combat this issue, multiple designs have been proposed for the accurate and reliable detection of stationary subjects with a PIR sensor. Initial designs utilize additional hardware with the inclusion of an optical shutter to periodically chop the FoV of the PIR sensor to artificially cause a motion change for the stationary human subject [18]. In addition, Ya Wang's group at Texas A&M has been awarded a one-million-dollar grant to enhance an optical shutter design for more reliable energy management solutions. The goal of the project is the development of an advanced, low-cost occupancy sensor named SLEEPIR that enhances industry PIR sensors for more accurate detection [19–24]. In our work, we propose two varying systems for stationary human subject detection using a PIR sensor. MI-PIR, the first design, classifies room occupancy through a 36 s rotation to induce the motion necessary for human detection. CM-PIR, on the other hand, relies on the chest motion from the heart to detect stationary subjects. These two designs will be presented further throughout this chapter.

2.2 *AI*

AI refers to the use of a computer to mimic human knowledge. The origin of AI can be traced to the 1950s, but overall, the field of AI is still premature [25]. Machine learning (ML) is a subset of AI and refers to a computer's ability to train itself without being explicitly told how to do so. DL is a subset of ML and is referred to as a type of neural network, one that trains itself through multilayered networks of data operation [26]. DL is an immensely powerful tool that can automatically learn from unstructured datasets, learning the slight variations that exist between the data samples while functioning like the neurons in the brain. AI is consistently used with non-contact ambient sensors to learn from the complex scenarios that exist withing these datasets. There exist various algorithms utilized for this purpose including ML algorithms such as Random Forest, Support Vector Machine, and Gaussian process regression (GPR) and DL algorithms including artificial neural networks (ANN), recurrent neural networks (RNN), and convolutional neural networks (CNN). In our work, we utilize GPR for precise indoor localization and ANN, RNN, and CNN as comparison for each other classification.

A Gaussian process can be completely defined by its mean and covariance function and is defined as a collection of random variables, with any finite number of which have (consistent) joint Gaussian distributions. GPRs remain powerful tools due to its probabilistic methods of predicting the output mean and variance conditional on a specific input at a specific instance of time. GPR models differ from classification models in that a location estimation can be predicted from GPR models, whereas a classification algorithm outputs classification results. Various parameters in the implementation of these models are to be optimized, including the kernel function [27]. There exist a variety of kernels that are often used in implementation of GPR models including Squared Exponential, Periodic, and Matern, just to name a few [28]. Performance of these models are often indicated with the quantification of the mean squared error (MSE) which is shown in Eq. (2). y_j refers to the observed values, $y(x_j)$ refers to the predicted values, and N is the number of data points in the training set [15].

$$MSE = \frac{1}{N}\sum_{j=1}^{N}\left(y_j - y\left(x_j\right)\right)^2 \tag{2}$$

In terms of DL, ANNs are the most basic feedforward approaches to learning and are used for a variety of tasks including pattern recognition, image recognition, and natural language processing. ANNs are composed of multiple dense layers that feedforward and do not learn recursively [29]. RNNs, on the other hand, are a recursive approach to learning, having an internal memory and making them particularly useful for time-series data classifications. RNNs work by taking time and sequence into account, where the output of one layer will in turn be fed to the input of a previous layer [30]. This approach to learning suffers from the vanishing gradient issue and must be overcome with the use of long-short term memory (LSTM) units in the application [31]. CNNs are often utilized for image recognition tasks as their architecture is designed specifically for this purpose. CNNs consist of multiple layers including fully connected layers, max pooling layers, convolutional and non-linearity layers [29].

Adequate reporting of these algorithms is essential, and the metric used for performance measurement often varies based on the classification task at hand.

Broadly, Explainable AI is a new field that is based on assessing the performance of ML algorithms to alleviate the black-box stigma surrounding AI [32, 33]. In general cases, reporting of the performance is completed with metrics such as accuracy, F1 score, area-under-the-curve, precision, or recall. Accuracy refers to the number of correct predictions that the statistical modeling labeled correctly divided by the total number of predictions that were made. Classification reports are often presented as a table that includes accuracy and various additional metrics. Visually, reporting of the confusion matrices, visual data, and training and testing curves also aids in the understanding of the performance. Confusion matrices visually identify the true positive (TP), true negative (TN), false positive (FP), and false negative (FN) of each classification by presenting the number of testing samples that were correctly and incorrectly classified. The confusion matrix provides actual values and expected values on the axes, and the resulting internal values are indicative of the number of correctly labeled samples in either normalized or unnormalized form. For the purposes of human detection and biometric authentication, we primarily rely on accuracy, visual data, classification reports, and confusion matrices to present the performance of the algorithms used.

2.3 Human Monitoring

There exist various methodologies for human monitoring purposes using ambient sensors and AI in related work. Ambient sensor modalities in literature that have been utilized for human monitoring purposes include microwave sensors, thermal sensors, and optical sensors. In terms of utilizing microwave sensors for human monitoring purposes, multiple sensors were distributed in the environment for multi-person HAR using a 3D-CNN for learning [34]. Using solely ambient thermal sensors and ML algorithms, detection of human presence was shown to be 100% accurate, with additional classifications of occupancy count estimation and HAR proving 100 and 97.5% accurate, respectively. The position of the thermal sensors affected the results of this work, with three sensors being deployed in this work, each having a horizontal FoV of 125° ([35]). An infrared active imaging system and a CNN learning model were utilized for human detection with a specific application to instances of home fires in another related work [36]. Further, image sensors were deployed iteratively for occupancy counts in a large exhibition hall with optical sensors deployed at entrances and exits. Learning of the occupancy counts in each zone of the exhibition hall was accomplished with an RNN with LSTM units [37].

Worth mentioning are the commonality of utilizing ambient signals for human monitoring purposes. In terms of leveraging ambient signals for human monitoring purposes, related works have utilized passive radio frequency identification (RFID) tags, passive RF signals, active RF signals, and Wi-Fi CSI. For example, a *SmartWall* composed of multiple passive RFID tags were utilized for localization and HAR purposes [38]. Similar in usage of passive RF-based signals, our group has published work on utilizing passive RF signals for human detection in residential and automobile environments. This work utilizes principal component analysis (PCA) for dimensionality reduction, recursive feature elimination with logistic regression, and ML algorithms for accurate human detection [39]. More common in literature are the use of active band RF signals for human monitoring applications. State-of-the-art research performed by the MIT CSAIL group has shown the efficacy of such approach, through the classification of human activities and their respective locations even through walls and occlusions [40–42]. Further, a millimeter-wave radar system was proposed for its low-cost approach in the proposed *RadHAR* system for HAR of five different exercise activities using a CNN-LSTM learning model [43]. Wi-Fi CSI via IoT devices can also prove successful at human monitoring, for HAR was shown to achieve 97.6% accuracy using a novel DL framework which was coined AE-LRCN [44].

In addition to the success of the previously mentioned sensor modalities, PIR sensors also have proven successful in human monitoring applications. Through a sensor fusion of PIR sensors and camera modalities, *HeteroSense* obtained accurate classifications for presence, occupancy count, trajectory or tracking, and basic multiclass activity recognition [45]. In *HeteroSense,* stereo-vision cameras are placed at entrances and multiple PIR sensors are deployed throughout the indoor environment for accurate classification. Sensor fusion with PIR sensors is popular in human monitoring applications, as the binary output of the PIR sensor is used for trajectory detection of the human subject and the other sensor modality is traditionally used for more continuous monitoring in sedentary moments. Another sensor fusion system can be seen with a geriatric monitoring application utilizing eight PIR sensors in a mock apartment environment with one wearable device connected to the thigh of the monitored subject. In this instance, a Bayesian particle filtering sensor fusion algorithm is applied for greater indoor localization accuracy [46]. In a similar sense, PIR sensors were deployed for early detection of dementia based on classification of travel patterns with a CNN learning model [47]. In terms of HAR using only PIR sensors, in the proposed system *ALPAS,* four activities completed on a sofa were classified with a F-measure of 57% using only two analog PIR sensors [48].

Although indoor localization has been classified through DL algorithms, indoor localization via GPR models is a common approach to localization. Regression is seen as superior in terms of indoor localization as estimation of testing data can apply to new coordinate systems in the environment of interest. One example of such an approach for indoor localization is coined *DeepMap*, a deep Gaussian process for indoor radio map construction and indoor localization [49]. The received signal strength (RSS) of Wi-Fi signals are used as fingerprints in this related work, for which the deep Gaussian process is fed and learns from these RSS values and their respective coordinates for accurate human localization. Similarly, authors in related work utilized Wi-Fi received signal strength indicator (RSSI) fingerprinting data for indoor localization via GPR, in which a CNN was also deployed to learn the features from RSSI data before being fed into the GPR model. The RSSI fingerprints were pre-processed in this case to represent images, in which such a designed process in this work of CNN + GPR with a Matern kernel proved superior to the k-

Nearest Neighbor algorithm in compared work [50]. A novel multi-person tracking framework was proposed utilizing a GPR observation model through a transfer learning approach. The prediction from the Kalman Filter feeds into the GPR model to estimate the targets' location and then the output of the GPR model is then used as the measurement input into the Kalman Filter [51]. In a work completed by our research group, the offline training phase is modeled by a 3D point cloud and the developed GPR model learns from the RSS of Wi-Fi signals for matching completed during the online stage. This methodology proved accurate for indoor localization on an iOS platform [52].

For elderly monitoring, indoor localization and HAR are two applications that significantly aid in greater independence for the monitored person. The caregiver and hospital system will be able to check on the status of the aging individual and monitor potentially harmful activities without being physically in their presence. Common in many systems designed specifically for the elderly and neurodegenerative populations is the detection of fall events, as fall events are the leading cause of death in these populations [53]. Many fall detection systems rely on sensors embedded in wearable devices for accurate detection of fall events, yet there exist ambient sensing systems that are designed for accurate classification of fall events. One such instance is proposed where the authors used a video-based detection system [54]. Human poses in this related work are used as features that are fed into a CNN for feature extraction and classification, achieving high sensitivity and specificity in comparison to other fall detection systems using raw RGB data. In neurodegenerative monitoring, an ultra-low-power radio signal device coined *Emerald* was developed and subsequently monitored seven PD patients passively with a focus on gait, home activity, and time in bed [55].

With the presentation of related systems based on ambient sensors and statistical learning algorithms, one can determine the shortcomings in these various systems. For example, those systems that rely on video-based detection are prone to privacy concerns that limit its long-term usage in at-home monitoring systems. In addition, video-based systems can be expensive for widespread deployment in assistive care facilities. Some systems with active sensors are prone to health and energy concerns, such as in the case of active RF signals. Some systems that deploy specific sensors, or PIR sensors in the traditional sense, are limited by the small FoV, requiring multiple sensors deployed in the monitored environment. Terminal devices used in sensor fusion with PIR sensors require the user to remember to consistently wear the device, causing intrusion on the monitored human subject. Therefore, as mentioned, there exists a need for inexpensive, non-intrusive, accurate, and expanded ambient sensing systems towards the reliable monitoring of aging individuals. A PIR sensor that extends the FoV to monitor an entire environment and accurately detect stationary human subjects could potentially fill the gaps in this related work.

2.4 Biometric Authentication

Biometric authentication methodologies vary in the modality and the metric used for classification. For instance, wearable devices have utilized biometric authentication methodologies towards the goal of secure and implicit authentication of these devices. One instance of this was presented with the usage of hybrid biometrics for biometric authentication, using calorie burn and metabolic equivalent of task (MET) metrics during sedentary and non-sedentary stages [56]. In terms of ambient, non-contact sensing for authentication purposes, many systems rely on camera modalities, such as in the case of imaging of fingernail plates and finger knuckles. Utilizing rank-level fusion of the two image features, the proposed system achieved 100% accuracy from a database containing 890 total images of 178 volunteers [57]. These examples highlight the variations in methodologies for the common biometric authentication goal. Towards biometric authentication systems that are less prone to forgery and indicate living human presence, heart-related biometrics have garnered much attention in recent years.

Electrocardiogram (ECG) is a measurement of the electrical activity of the heart, which is generally dependent on surface electrodes. The waveforms that exist in an ECG signal include the P, Q, R, S, and T waves, which are indicative of repolarization and depolarization of various parts of the heart [15, 58]. These collected ECG signals are commonly deployed for biometric identification and biometric authentication purposes based on the unique QRS complex that exists for each heartbeat of the ECG signal. More generally, these methods for biometric identification and authentication are based on the physiological background that everyone has a unique heartbeat due to the variations in opening and closing of valves and varying sizes and shapes of each heart. Common methodologies for biometric authentication and identification with ECG signals rely on DL to learn the slight variations that often exist between the QRS complexes. For example, a CNN was deployed to intrinsically learn the features contained within the MIT-BIH database of ECG signal data resulting in a 99% accurate biometric identification system. The novelty of this proposed system is such that this methodology eliminates the usual time-extensive manual feature engineering process [59]. Likewise, another biometric identification system based on ECG signal data was proposed, where in this instance, the novelty was based on the QRS-resampling strategy that was proposed to handle the variations in heart rate. This QRS-resampling strategy with a PCANet DL architecture allowed for a 94.4% accurate identification system that is robust to heart rate variability [60]. Towards the goal of improving the generalization ability of ECG identification systems, a cascaded CNN was proposed for biometric identification of ECG signal data in another related work, where the F-CNN is used for feature extraction and M-CNN is used for classification [61]. Although accurate enough to identify every individual included in the dataset, ECG signals require contact with the user and are reliant on expensive hardware. To improve biometric systems for everyday usage, such as in the case of IoT, capturing heart-related signals with more advantageous sensor modalities is examined.

Collecting an accurate and informative heart rate signal is more difficult with non-contact sensors. A few solutions, however, have been proposed in recent years on this topic. ECG signals can now be captured via wearable devices such as an Apple Watch or in the case of capacitive coupled electrodes embedded within clothing. In the latter example, the researchers proposed methods for artifact reduction in such non-contact ECG monitoring examples, showing that their proposed empirical wavelet transform with traditional wavelet transform approach was successful at reducing motion artifacts and restoring the QRS complexes [62]. Moreover, the breathing pattern and respiratory rate (RR) has been shown to be accurately quantified via RGB cameras [63]. Collecting these signals would allow for a non-contact, heart-related biometric system; yet, collecting RGB images raises privacy issues that should be avoided for a long-term monitoring solution. In more recent work, the WiFi CSI ambient signals have shown success at estimating the RR through high-resolution spectrogram-based CSI features for a COVID-19 monitoring application [64]. A PIR sensor would address the shortcomings of other sensor systems and fit the needs of a long-term monitoring solution. Presented in related work is a PIR sensor that accurately estimates the resting heart of 30 subjects using a novel acceleration filter that is presented in Eq. (3) [65]. The magnitude of the heart-rate signal is much greater than the respiratory signal for the applied acceleration filter, allowing for accurate resting heart rate estimation from a PIR sensor in this related work. The novel acceleration filter in Eq. (3) computes the second derivative with a convolving triangular window and simple Lagrange low pass filter to the raw PIR analog sensor data.

$$g_2' = [1\ 4\ 4 - 4 - 10 - 4\ 4\ 4\ 1] \tag{3}$$

This acceleration filter in Eq. (3) is utilized and included as a feature for biometric authentication in our work. In their methodology, subjects sat 1 m away from the PIR sensor while remaining motionless, and their chest motion was collected at a 10 Hz sampling rate [65]. Showing to be successful at extracting the heart rate of individuals with a PIR sensor, we follow a similar methodology in our CM-PIR system. In comparison to a proposed system using a PIR sensor for biometric authentication, a system coined *Cardiac Scan* utilizes a DC-coupled continuous-wave radar for the authentication of 78 subjects at one common location. The cardiac motion acts as a biometric in this case, showing to be 98.61% accurate using a SVM algorithm with RBF kernel [66]. This non-contact biometric authentication system for an IoT device indicates the similarity to our proposed CM-PIR system.

3 Motion Induced PIR

MI-PIR was previously introduced as a novel method for stationary human presence detection using one analog PIR sensor and an ANN DL model [13]. Additionally, MI-PIR consists of a robotic actuator, a platform, a thermal insulator, a microcontroller, and a PC. The complete set-up of MI-PIR is included in Fig. 1(b). The thermal insulator is made of cardboard, as this material was shown to accurately block the infrared radiation detected from the movement of the robotic actuator. A more long-term material will be developed and replace the cardboard in this system in a future model. The thermal insulator sits on the platform and subsequently the robotic actuator. The robotic actuator used in the MI-PIR design is the Dynamixel MX-28, while the platform is a Hokuyo UTM-30LX-EW which serves no other purpose than to be used as a flat surface for the thermal insulation material. The Elegoo Uno R3 microcontroller connects to the Panasonic AMN24112 PIR sensor for data conversion and transmission to the PC. This full MI-PIR design classifies a room occupancy and related parameters every 36 s due to the 26 s forward motion and the 10 s backward motion to complete one full cycle.

In our initial work, MI-PIR was extended to classify three additional occupancy parameters on top of stationary human presence detection, which included occupancy count estimation, relative location classification, and human target differentiation. New in this work is the addition of precise indoor localization and HAR in both an office environment and residential environment. We utilize a GPR model for precise indoor localization achieving 493.7 cm^2 MSE in an office environment with multiple users and 426.4 cm^2 MSE for Student 1 only of Table 1. An RNN model with LSTM units for HAR achieved 100% accuracy in the office environment for classifying activities of Student 1 only. In the residential environment, the GPR model achieved 131.4 cm^2 MSE for precise indoor localization of one individual and the RNN architecture achieved 98% accuracy between six total labels for HAR. The data collection, pre-processing, and results of the MI-PIR system will be fully addressed in this section.

3.1 Ambient Environments

The office location is in Dodge Hall, an academic office building on the campus of Oakland University in Rochester, Michigan, USA. This office location consists of five different PC locations labeled as "Location (L1)" through "Location 5 (L5)", where MI-PIR is placed for data collection at Location 1. In addition, the office location is split into three different walking paths for HAR data collection. The office location is 5.18 m in length and 3.96 m in width and is only accessible by key access. As a result, student researchers are of those with access and are commonly using the office space. Each researcher in the lab has a common workstation, but due to fluidity in the student researchers, there does exist some variation in the student locations. The office location has been modeled and is presented below in Fig. 2. L1 through L5 label the locations of student researchers and W1 through W3 label walking paths in this figure.

In relation to the office location, a residential location is more indicative of an elderly monitoring situation, and thus the MI-PIR system was additionally tested in an apartment bedroom. The residential environment is 4.57 m in length and

Table 1 MI-PIR data collection in the office space location for each of the five classifications and two regression models. The number label used for DL, along with the real label and available samples for a 36 s rotation time is included

Classification	Number label for ML	Real label	Available samples
Room classification	0	Unoccupied	854
	1	Occupied	2803
Occupancy count estimation	0	No people	854
	1	One person	1936
	2	Two people	702
	3	Three people	165
Relative location classification	0	Unoccupied	854
	1	Location 1	174
	2	Location 2	1240
	3	Location 3	153
	4	Location 4	369
	6	Locations 1 and 2	105
	10	Locations 2 and 3	44
	11	Locations 2 and 4	100
	12	Locations 2 and 5	250
	15	Locations 4 and 5	203
	23	Locations 2, 3, and 5	138
	24	Locations 3, 4, and 5	21
	25	Locations 2, 4, and 5	6
Human target differentiation	0	Unoccupied	854
	1	Student 1	1936
	2	Students 1 and 2	32
	3	Students 1 and 3	181
	4	Students 1 and 4	386
	5	Students 1 and 5	103
	6	Students 1, 4, and 5	98
	7	Students 1, 3, and 5	46
	8	Students 1, 4, and 6	21
Indoor localization	(250, 10)	Unoccupied	7136
	(415, 70)	Location 1	279
	(415, 265)	Location 2	1883
	(250, 265)	Location 3	356
	(80, 265)	Location 4	699
	(50, 60)	Location 5	618
Indoor localization—Student 1	(415, 70)	Location 1	174

(continued)

Table 1 (continued)

Classification	Number label for ML	Real label	Available samples
	(415, 265)	Location 2	483
	(250, 265)	Location 3	153
	(80, 265)	Location 4	369
Activity recognition—Student 1	0	Unoccupied	191
	1	Sitting	102
	2	Walking	101

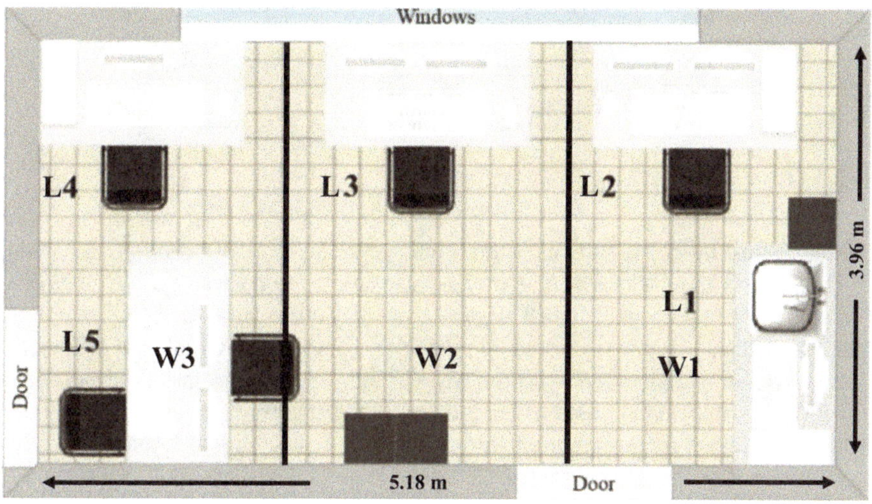

Fig. 2 The model of the office space. "L1" through "L5" indicate the five stationary locations in the office space and "W1" through "W3" indicate the three walking paths during the HAR data collection. MI-PIR is located on the counter at L1

3.65 m in width, just smaller than that of the office environment. In this location, a relative location classification and HAR classification are completed. In addition, a precise indoor localization is applied to identify the results of estimating a human occupant's position in a residential environment. This specific residential environment is modeled in Fig. 3. This apartment model indicates the locations for which each activity is completed, specifically presenting Activity 1 ("A1") of "Working at the Desk" at Location 2 ("L2") in Fig. 3. Further, Location 1 on Fig. 3 ("L1") indicates the locations of Activity 2 ("A2") and Activity 3 ("A3"), "Laying on the Ground" and "Exercising on the Ground", respectively. Location 3 is located at the bed for which Activity 4 ("A4") and Activity 5 ("A5") are completed of "Watching TV on Bed" and "Sleeping on Bed", respectively.

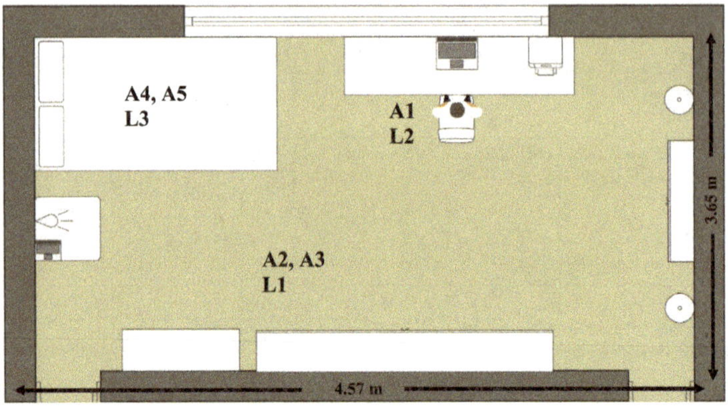

Fig. 3 Model of residential environment data collection. MI-PIR is located next to the bed, indicated by the outward signals

3.2 *Data Acquisition*

For data acquisition, MI-PIR scans the room every 36 s in a 130° motion, including both a forward and backward trajectory. As a result, the horizontal FoV is increased from 93 to 223° with the MI-PIR design. Data was collected at a 10 Hz sampling rate. Each data sample is synced to match the ambient environment e.g., each data collection sample starts with the MI-PIR system pointing in the farthest east direction. For unoccupied data collection, an additional 36 s is included to copy the data that matches the accurate situation. The data collected was copied from the serial monitor of the Arduino integrated development environment (IDE) and then converted to a CSV format, where it was cleaned and manually labeled. Each data sample includes the labels for learning and the time for each classification. The data samples are finally sent to their respective folders for each classification.

3.2.1 Office Environment

Office data collection for stationary human presence detection, occupancy count estimation, relative location classification, and human target differentiation was completed between August to December of 2019. This covered the change in the summer semester to the fall semester on campus, allowing for variations in the student researchers and their usual locations in the office environment. The ambient environment in the data collection varied due to the sunlight changes between seasons that existed with the open windows in the office. These changes between locations and ambient environments allow for a more robust monitoring system. Precise indoor localization via GPR is based on the same data collection; however, data collection for the "walking" label of HAR was collected in March by Student 1. HAR in this office environment is completed with Student 1 only and precise indoor localization is presented with a Student 1 only model and with a full data collection model.

In terms of the office environment, the room occupants are not aware of the data collection process while its ongoing, allowing for a data collection process that is more representative of the workday. Data collection is a continuous process until the room state is changed e.g., a room occupant stands up, changes seat location, leaves the room, etc. In that case, Student 1 who runs the data collection process, starts a new continuous data sample. Overall, Student 1 ensures the data collection process is accurate, as this student participates in each of the data collection samples. In terms of the unoccupied scenarios, Student 1 remains outside the office door, ensuring no student researcher or other university employee enters the office during this process. For the "walking" scenarios, Student 1 walked continuously in three different specified paths as included in Fig. 2. W1 refers to the first specified location for a continuous pacing path, W2 is the second, and W3 is the last. All classifications include the recorded "sitting" samples of all the students, whereas the "walking" samples of Student 1 were included for the HAR classification only.

For indoor localization, more unoccupied slots are appended to match the number of coordinates presented in a three-person example that is needed for ML. For example, a data sample of Location 1 and Location 3 would include the coordinates "(415, 70), (250, 265), (250, 10)", as the third person is not present in the data collection process. Data for all six classifications (room classification, occupancy count estimation, relative location classification, human target differentiation, precise indoor localization, and HAR) is presented in Table 1. This table includes the number label or coordinate system used for ML, the actual label, and the number of 36 s samples for each label.

3.2.2 Residential Environment

Residential data collection was completed by Student 1 only for five different activities and one unoccupied scenario. As Student 1 is the only occupant for data collection, the subject knows data collection is ongoing in this case. The full complete breakdown of data collection for relative location classification, HAR, and precise indoor localization in the residential environment is included in Table 2. The five activities and their integer labels for ML are included in this table, with the addition of the coordinate system based on the activity completed. The locations are not provided the coordinate system in this case, as the activities differentiated slightly at the precise location. The unoccupied scenario was given a coordinate system close to the entrance door, like that of the office environment indoor localization. Multiple activities are completed at the same location as to prove that the system is not dependent on location for classification e.g., two activities at the same location can be differentiated based on the motion of the subject. Activity 3 of "Laying on the Ground" was included in the dataset as an activity representative of a possible fall in the geriatric population. In this instance, Student 1 remains motionless on the ground throughout the continuous data sample collection. All activities in the dataset for the residential environment are completed continuously, where each activity is roughly 2 h of data with at most three continuous data samples for each activity.

3.3 Data Pre-processing

Collected data from MI-PIR was pre-processed in Jupyter Notebook using Python. To increase the data samples and allow for quicker classification times, continuous data samples were batched into 360 s samples based on the time data included in the CSV file. The 360 s time window accounts for a 36 s complete cycle at a 10 Hz sampling rate. Those that were less than 360 s samples at the end of the continuous data sample were deleted. These 360 s samples were then ready to be used in feature extraction. In total, there exists 3657 samples for the first four classifications included in Table 1, 10,971 for precise indoor localization of the full data collection model due to the splitting of individual labels and the appending of unoccupied scenarios, 1179 for precise indoor localization of Student 1, and 394 samples for the HAR classification of Student 1. For the residential environment, there are 1147 samples to be utilized for training and testing. The full complete breakdown of data collection for relative location classification, HAR, and precise indoor localization in the residential environment is included in Table 2. Data for each classification in each environment is split into 70% training, 15% testing, and 15% validation for learning purposes.

Table 2 Data collection for the MI-PIR system in a residential environment. Locations, coordinates, and activities with their integer labels used for ML and DL are presented

Classification	Number label for ML	Real label	Available samples
Relative location classification	0	Unoccupied	185
	1	Location 1	370
	2	Location 2	208
	3	Location 3	384
Indoor localization	(425, 50)	Unoccupied	185
	(290, 260)	Working at desk	208
	(225, 150)	Laying on ground	186
	(200, 150)	Exercise on ground	184
	(125, 260)	Watch TV on bed	174
	(100, 270)	Sleep on bed	210
Activity recognition	0	Unoccupied	185
	1	Working at desk	208
	2	Laying on ground	186
	3	Exercise on ground	184
	4	Watch TV on bed	174
	5	Sleep on bed	210

Through various feature experimentations, the signal power of the time-series raw MI-PIR analog voltage was found to be the most indicative of human presence. The signal power of the raw voltage was taken for each 360 s time window, where the absolute value of the fast Fourier transform (FFT) allowed for this calculation to be completed. This calculation was also completed with Python in the Jupyter Notebook. Other experimented features include discrete wavelet transform (DWT), raw voltage, and a standard deviation statistical feature, but all of which proved poor in stationary human presence detection using an ANN. Further, statistical testing of stationary human presence proved inadequate due to the multiple ambient environments collected over the multiple seasons in the office environment. The signal power not only achieved high accuracy for room occupancy, but for each of the other classifications. The signal power feature vector is normalized from 0 to 1 using min max normalization of the sklearn package before being used for many of the classifications. The GPR model performed better with the raw signal power, and in some cases the raw signal power showed better results in the neural networks, such as in the case of the maximum sensing distance quantification that will be presented later. Overall, the raw signal power and the normalized signal power are both used in the statistical learning models developed for the MI-PIR system.

3.4 AI

Four different models have been developed for MI-PIR related classifications. As mentioned, these models include three DL algorithms and one ML algorithm. An ANN, RNN, and CNN were all utilized for the four original occupancy parameters as comparison to identify the maximum accuracy obtained between the three neural networks. The GPR model is utilized for precise indoor localization. The most accurate neural network architecture will be utilized for the HAR classifications between both environments. All models in this work were built with the Keras DL framework in Python.

The ANN architectures used differ with the classification due to the number of classes outputted. For example, the human target differentiation requires eight classes, and the room occupancy classification parameter is only a binary classification which requires two classes. With that, room occupancy classification utilizes the binary crossentropy function as the loss function, and the other three parameters utilize the sparse categorical crossentropy function as the loss function. The room classification also differs in the fact that it utilizes the stochastic gradient descent (sgd) optimizer, whereas the other four classifications utilize the Adam optimizer. In general, the ANN model is composed of an input layer, a hidden layer, and output layer with multiple variations in the dimensions of each due to the number of classification output labels that are needed. For example, the ANN model for room classification of binary output consists of two dimensions for the input layer, two for the hidden layer, and one for the output layer. For an extensive table highlighting the architectures of each ANN model used for room classification, occupancy count

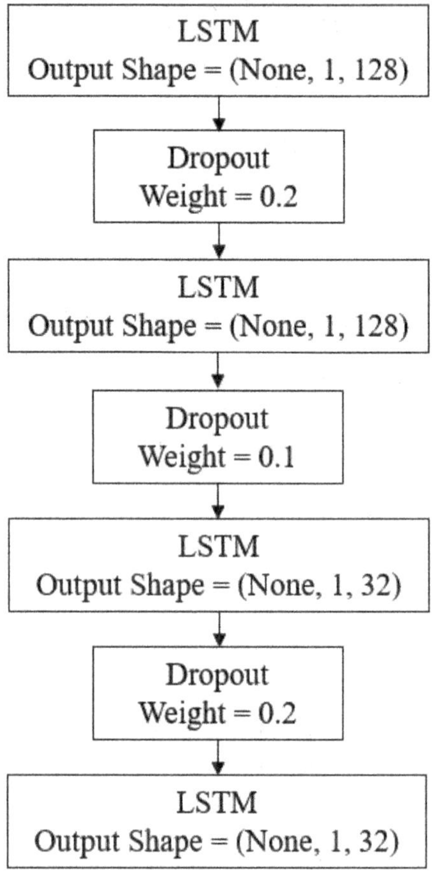

Fig. 4 The RNN architecture utilized for the HAR classification in the office environment. The other RNN architectures used in this work follow a similar structure with varying output shapes due to the variation in classification

estimation, relative location classification, and human target differentiation, we direct the reader to our previous work [13].

The RNN model developed consists of two LSTM units, two dense layers, and three dropout layers to aid in overfitting of the models. The LSTM units consist of 128 dimensions, the dense layers of 32 for all but the output layer of the binary classification in which a dimension of 2 is utilized, and the dropout layers utilize 0.2 and 0.1 weights. Rectified linear unit (ReLu) and softmax are utilized for activation functions, where softmax is used as the output activation function. The Adam optimization function and sparse categorical crossentropy function are utilized for all four original models. Figure 4 presents the RNN architecture used for the HAR classification, however, the other RNN architectures used follow a similar structure. All original four occupancy classifications use 100 epochs for learning, whereas the RNN model for HAR classification uses 50 epochs.

The CNN developed includes two convolution layers, one dropout layer, one max pooling layer, and two dense layers. The convolutional layers use filters of 64 and kernel size of 3, the one dropout layers uses a weight of 0.5, max pooling layer uses a pool size of 2, and the dense layers consists of one that is 100 dimensions, and the output dense layer is the dimension of the number of labels. The relu and softmax activation functions are utilized similarly for the CNN model. Sparse categorical crossentropy is utilized for the loss function of these models and Adam is used as the optimizer function. 10 epochs are used for the CNN.

The GPR model utilized for precise indoor localization is developed with the sklearn package in Python. The MSE output of the GPR model was compared with three different kernels: Matern, RBF, and ExpSineSquared. The Matern kernel showed the best result and is thus utilized for the precise indoor localization regression problems in this work.

3.5 Occupancy Parameter Classification

The classification reports for the four original occupancy parameters using an ANN in the office environment (room occupancy, occupancy count estimation, relative location classification, and human target differentiation) were reported in our previous work [13]. The room classification occupancy parameter for detecting human presence in an office environment achieved 99% accuracy. The occupancy count estimation of differentiating between no people and, at maximum, three people achieved 91% accuracy. Relative location classification at differentiating between Location 1 through Location 5, with multiple combinations, achieved 92%. Finally, human target differentiation of eight different combinations of people with an unoccupied scenario achieved 93%.

For relative location classification in the residential environment, we used the developed RNN DL model to achieve 98% accuracy. With three locations and a constant human subject present, Student 1, the relative location classification was less complex than that in the office location. However, for an elderly monitoring system, it is imperative to know the location of the elderly individual in a non-intrusive and passive manner. The location of the elderly individual can provide peace of mind to the caregiver through the monitoring system. As such, this classification is still essential to report towards the goal of an accurate geriatric monitoring solution.

3.6 Expanding MI-PIR

Before applying the MI-PIR system to precise indoor localization and HAR, we aimed to optimize and quantify the parameters of the MI-PIR system. These metrics include the selection of an optimal DL architecture, optimal rotation time, and maximum sensing distance. From the results, the RNN model and 36 s rotation time are found to be the optimal DL model and rotation time, respectively. From the maximum sensing distance quantification, MI-PIR can accurately detect stationary and non-stationary subjects up to 21 m. The complete results of this expansion are included below.

3.6.1 Optimization

In the hopes of a quicker classification time, the optimal rotation time for classification of the room occupancy parameters in the office environment was experimented with. Three different classification times were addressed for comparison. These include 36 s for a complete rotation of the robotic actuator, 26 s for the front scan only, and 10 s for the backward scan only. This analysis was completed within the developed Python code, where the batches were first developed for the 36 s rotation time. Following, the last 10 s would be removed for the 26 s examination and vice versa for the 26 s classification. Thirty-six seconds proved to be the most accurate of the three times, and despite the additional time required, the relatively large increase in accuracy outweighs the additional classification time. The results of this optimization are included in Table 3 with reported accuracies from the previously developed ANN.

The RNN and CNN introduced in this section were developed to compare the reported accuracies from the ANN to more sophisticated models. The results of this optimization are also presented in Table 3 for each of the four occupancy parameters in the office environment. From these results, the RNN is shown to be the most accurate DL model for MI-PIR, as indicated by the maximum accuracy obtained for each of the occupancy classifications. The RNN performing the best in these four classifications is expected due to the time-series nature of the input data. The RNN model will be utilized for the rest of the work due to these results.

3.6.2 Quantification

Utilizing the RNN DL model, we aimed to quantify the maximum sensing distance for possible extension of the design to larger environments. In addition, this metric would allow for better comparison to existing human monitoring systems. In this experiment, we collected data of Student 1 walking and standing at iterative linear distances away from the MI-PIR system in three different ambient environments: a residential hallway, a construction warehouse, and a gymnasium. Three ambient environments were included as there was a need for greater distance away from the sensor following the results of each environment. In the residential environment, data was collected for an unoccupied scenario and from 1 to 12 m away from the MI-PIR system. In the construction warehouse, data was collected for an unoccupied scenario and 13 through 19 m away from MI-PIR at 1 m increments. In the gymnasium, data was collected for an unoccupied scenario and distances at

Table 3 The results of the optimization of metrics used in the original MI-PIR system. The DL model and rotation time are optimized to advance the novel system

Optimization metric					
DL	Model	Room classification (%)	Occupancy count (%)	Location classification (%)	Human target differentiation (%)
	ANN	99	91	93	93
	RNN	100	93	95	94
	CNN	100	90	93	94
Rotation time	Time(s)	Room classification (%)	Occupancy count (%)	Location classification (%)	Human target differentiation (%)
	36	99	91	93	93
	26	98	84	84	89
	10	75	71	69	80

21, 41, and 43 m. For walking data collection in these environments, the human subject paced a few meters back and forth, whereas for stationary data collection, the human subject remained seated during the entirety of the collection. The maximum sensing distance for a stationary individual and moving individual was quantified by removing the data sample with the next farthest distance to quantify the RNN accuracy. The manufacturer lists the maximum sensing distance of the Panasonic AMN24112 PIR sensor as 10 m with the deployment of a PIR sensor in the traditional approach. The results of this maximum sensing quantification are compared between three different sample sets, one in which all the data is included, one of just motionless data, and one of just walking data. The results of this quantification are included in Table 4.

For each occupied scenario, about 3–5 min of data was collected with matching unoccupied scenarios at each ambient environment for balanced data. Therefore, in total, there exists 426 samples for maximum sensing distance quantification. With motion and motionless data combined, the maximum sensing distance for 100% accuracy was quantified as 41 m. With motionless data only, maximum sensing distance for 100% accuracy was found to be 21 m. Finally, for motion data only, the maximum sensing distance was also reported as 21 m.

From these reported results it is evident that MI-PIR has human detection capabilities beyond the reported 10 m distance reported by the manufacturer. The maximum sensing distance is quantified between three ambient environments, causing the DL model to learn from multiple locations. For more accurate maximum sensing quantification, data should be collected at one central location. The data collection and results of this work is more robust however, due to the multiple ambient environments. With the large jump between 21 to 41 m at the gymnasium location, the maximum sensing distance could be greater than the reported 21 m for stationary and non-stationary human subject detection. The 41 m maximum sensing distance quantification, which includes all the data, allows for learning of double the number of scenarios. With the additional training data, the distance of the monitored human subject is expanded. Verification of the maximum sensing distance will be addressed with additional data at the gymnasium location. With that being said, the MI-PIR system has shown to expand the sensing distance of the traditional analog PIR sensor to a recorded 21 m with motion and motionless data only, and even further with all the data included.

3.7 Precise Indoor Localization via GPR

The GPR model was applied for a regression method of indoor localization. The regression method, in comparison to the relative location classification, allows for estimation of the human occupant in comparison to the ground truth coordinate system. The coordinate system utilized for the precise indoor localization in the office environment is presented in Table 1. Two classifications are completed for the precise indoor localization in the office environment: one in which all stationary

Table 4 MI-PIR maximum sensing distance quantification of three different ambient environments using an RNN DL model. One subject sits and paces at iterative distances away from the sensor system for 3–5 min of continuous samples. The results present below indicate human detection sensing distance classification of including the farthest distance in the RNN DL model

Ambient environment	Environment type	Max. measured length (m)	Distance (m)	All data: Accuracy (%)	Motionless: Accuracy (%)	Motion: Accuracy (%)
Residential hallway	Rectangular hallway	12	1	100	100	100
			3	100	100	100
			7	100	100	100
			9	100	100	100
			10	100	100	100
			11	100	100	100
			12	100	100	100
Construction warehouse	Square facility	19	13	100	100	100
			14	100	100	100
			15	100	100	100
			16	100	100	100
			17	100	100	100
			18	100	100	100
			19	100	100	100
Gymnasium	Square gymnasium	47	21	100	100	100
			41	100	95	98
			43	95	91	95

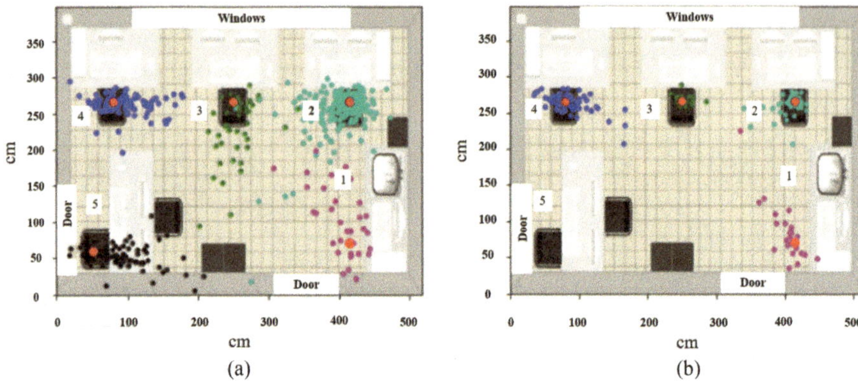

Fig. 5 Result of precise indoor localization using GPR with (**a**) all data (unoccupied result not shown) and (**b**) Subject A

data collected is utilized and another in which only the data from Student 1 is utilized. The Student 1 only model does not include data from Location 5 or any unoccupied data, whereas the model including all the data does include the unoccupied scenarios. Including two different regressions allows for a comparison of the models in learning from the signal power from multiple subjects in the office space to one in which there is only one person accounted for.

For multiple people, the MSE obtained is 493.7 cm^2. The accuracy of this model may be better represented visually. Figure 5(a) presents the accuracy of the model for precise indoor localization using a GPR model with a Matern kernel and with all the data collected for multiple variations in students present in the office environment. This model does not visually include the clustering of the unoccupied scenario, which is located near the door, as this data was only included as a means of balancing the data to match the coordinate systems of three people. With all the ground truth data for each location presented as red dots, and the estimations presented in varying colors, one can determine that the developed GPR model proved sufficient at clustering the testing data in their respective locations. With the Student 1 only model, on the other hand, the model produced a MSE of 426.4 cm^2. Although a better resulting MSE than the model with multiple people, the MSE is relatively similar. Also, based on the visual representation in Fig. 5(b), the clusters for the four respective locations of Student 1 are developed. The results of this work indicate that MI-PIR proves to not only classify locations in an office environment, but also estimate these locations in terms of coordinate systems. The exact coordinates of the students were not measured during training data and the student researchers were also free to subtly move their chairs. As a result, the MSE is not an exact indicator of the performance of these models, but rather this exercise proves to be a sufficient method for clustering of testing coordinates to the ground truth coordinate system. With more precise ground truth data, the MSE is hypothesized to decrease for both the full data collection method and for Student 1 only.

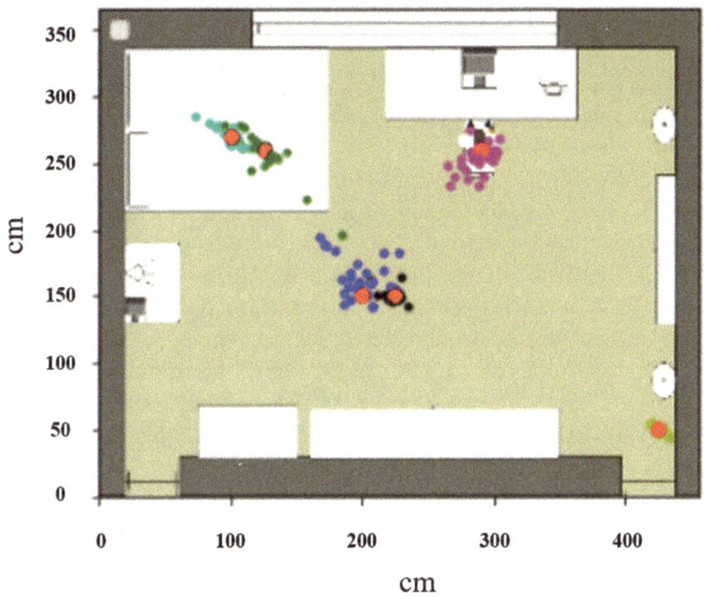

Fig. 6 GPR model of the residential environment, where each color represents a different activity. The yellow cluster near the entrance represents the unoccupied scenario

For precise indoor localization with a GPR model in the residential environment, the reported MSE is 131.4 cm^2. For better understanding of this reported metric, the modeled residential environment provides the clustering of the precise locations of each activity, as shown in Fig. 6. This model also proves accurate at clustering the locations of the activities. As a comparison, the GPR model can be more accurate in indoor localization as the estimation of future activities can be applied throughout the environment, whereas the classification of locations is either classified correctly or not. The unoccupied scenario is included in this visual display of the model, as indicated by the small yellow cluster close to the entrance door in Fig. 6.

3.8 HAR

As a proof of concept, a simple HAR classification model was developed for the office environment. Simple classification of sitting, walking, and an unoccupied scenario was hypothesized to show some level of indication that MI-PIR could accurately classify various activities in its FoV. The results of this classification would allow for expansion to a residential environment for a HAR system more indicative of the activities that an elderly individual would complete.

Student 1 data was only utilized in this classification. This data included stationary moments from the original data collection that was utilized in prior classification and regression problems. Specifically, this stationary data included samples from Location 2 and Location 4. In addition, this dataset includes walking sets from all the walking patterns: W1, W2, W3. In these instances, Student 1 paced for as long as 15 min, providing continuous data samples of walking data to classify. Overall, there exists 394 samples to be utilized for classification as presented in Table 1. With the 70%, 15%, 15% split of training, testing, and validation data that is completed in all the models referenced in this work, there exists 275 samples for training and 59 samples for testing.

The RNN model was utilized in this case for HAR classification in an office environment. The model proved 100% accurate at differentiating unoccupied, sitting, and walking scenarios completed by Student 1. The RNN proved its superiority with time-series data such as in the case of the normalized absolute value of the FFT. These results indicate that the MI-PIR system could prove accurate as a HAR system in a geriatric monitoring situation. To prove this hypothesis, MI-PIR was utilized in a residential environment for classification of additional activities.

Based on the success of the HAR classification in the office environment and towards the development of an elderly monitoring system, accurate HAR classification in a residential environment is an important task. With early success from differentiating walking from sitting in the office environment, this classification aims to extend the number of activities classified in a residential environment. The developed RNN model achieved 98% accuracy in this classification of five different activities and an unoccupied scenario. Two activities, "Exercising on Ground" and "Laying on Ground", were completed at Location 1, and two other activities, "Watching TV on Bed" and "Sleeping on Bed", were completed at Location 3. The model proves robust to differentiating activities at the same location, indicating that the variations in infrared radiation as indicated by the absolute value of the FFT are suitable for an accurate HAR model in a residential environment. The classification of the "Laying on Ground" label indicates the efficacy of detecting a potential fall event and classifying such activity in 36 s increments. This also would allow for greater state of mind of the caregiver in terms of an accurate elderly monitoring system. The accuracy of the RNN model utilized for this HAR classification is presented visually as a confusion matrix in Fig. 7. The integer labels provided on the confusion matrix correlate to the activities highlighted in Table 2. From this confusion matrix, one can identify high classification results, with only minimal confusion relating to the activity number label of "3" or real label of "Exercise on Ground".

4 Chest Motion PIR

MI-PIR was developed as a novel system for stationary human detection utilizing only one analog PIR sensor. Similarly, a system relying on the detection of the chest motion of a perfectly still stationary human subject for stationary human presence detection using one analog PIR sensor has been developed. This system is coined

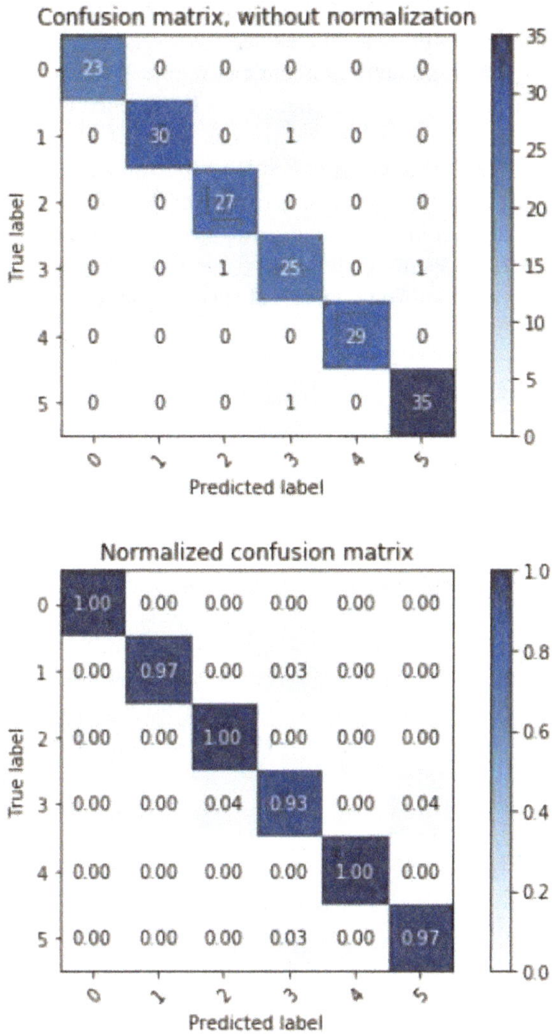

Fig. 7 Confusion matrix for HAR in the residential environment. The accuracy of HAR is reported as 98%, and the confusion matrix serves to highlight this reported accuracy. True labels and predicted labels are provided with integer labels that correspond to the activities provided in Table 2 for HAR in a residential environment

CM-PIR and has been previously presented in our past work [14]. CM-PIR consists of the Panasonic AMN24112 PIR sensor, an Elegoo Uno R3 microcontroller, a PC, and the RNN DL model for human detection and biometric authentication classification.

CM-PIR is based on the resting heart rate estimation using a PIR sensor methodology from related work, where the users are perfectly still 1 m away during the data collection process [65]. The filter to extract the heart rate from the individuals was presented in the introduction of this work in Eq. (3). Our first step in the human detection and biometric authentication process using CM-PIR was to verify the accuracy of the filter and estimating the human heart rate of individuals using a PIR sensor. After verifying this work with the heart rate monitor of the Apple Watch Series 3, we expanded the data collection process to include 16 subjects at nine different ambient environments. The accuracy of the model achieved 94% for human detection and 75% for biometric authentication of Subject A against all other potential adversaries. The results of this work are aimed to be utilized in a desk scenario, where the human subject can be detected and authenticated for security purposes at a 1-m distance.

4.1 Data Acquisition

CM-PIR successfully collected data for 16 subjects at nine different ambient locations. Each subject recorded data for at least 20 min, with many collecting for more trials and at various ambient environments. The subjects are of varying ages and sex, with the ages of the subjects ranging from 15 to 60 years old and six females and ten males included in the study. Some of the subjects utilized for the CM-PIR data collection are of family relation. In each ambient environment, the CM-PIR system would be set-up 1 m away on a surface that was on the chest level of the subject. The full data collection for the CM-PIR system is presented in Table 5.

4.2 Data Pre-processing

Upon data acquisition of 16 subjects at nine different locations, the data was pre-processed in Python. The overall CM-PIR flowchart is included in Fig. 8. In a similar manner to how the MI-PIR data was batched according to the rotation time, the CM-PIR data was batched to increase the number of data samples from the original data files. This involved identifying the optimal window size experimentally. The optimal window size was determined to be 90 s based on a balance between the number of available samples to learn from and the number of data points to be learned from. With the 90 s optimal selection in place, the next process was to apply a threshold to the raw PIR voltage data. In terms of a human subject in motion, the raw analog PIR voltage will spike from 5 V to 0 V as indicated by a sinusoidal swing. In terms of the early data collection of CM-PIR, the motion of the chest from a perfectly stationary human subject is between the ranges of 3 V to 2 V. To account for different ambient environments, a threshold of 3.5 V to 1.5 V was applied to the 90 s batches. If there are any data points greater than 3.5 V or less than 1.5 V in the sample, that 90 s batch would be removed. As a result, Table 5 indicates the available samples from the collected samples after the threshold was applied. With the threshold, four

Table 5 Data collection for the CM-PIR system including the data distribution for stationary detection, biometric authentication, and overall subject distribution. The data included is for a 90 s window size and 3.5 to 1.5 V threshold that reduced the number of available samples from collected to used

Category	Data collected (samples)	Data used (samples)	Integer label	Real label	Location
Stationary detection	123	122	0	Unoccupied	A-D
	443	295	1	Occupied	A-I
Biometric authentication	123	122	0	Unoccupied	A-D
	219	133	1	Subject A	A-D
	224	162	2	Adversaries	B, D-I
Individual subject distribution	123	122	0	Unoccupied	A-D
	219	133	1	Subject A	A-D
	40	34	2	Subject B	A-C
	19	19	3	Subject C	B
	35	32	4	Subject D	B
	18	14	5	Subject E	E
	9	7	6	Subject F	E
	11	11	7	Subject G	B
	6	0	8	Subject H	F
	14	0	9	Subject I	G
	13	11	10	Subject J	G
	12	6	11	Subject K	B
	7	0	12	Subject L	H
	12	0	13	Subject M	I
	13	11	14	Subject N	F
	12	7	15	Subject O	F
	13	10	16	Subject P	D

human subjects and three ambient environments were completely removed from the dataset. As a result, CM-PIR would then detect and classify 12 subjects and an unoccupied scenario from six different ambient environments.

Following both the window size selection and applied threshold, feature calculations were then made on this data. As indicated by the MI-PIR system, the absolute value of the FFT proved to be an accurate feature for human presence and related occupancy parameters. This feature was used for the CM-PIR data, as a result. Indicated in orange in Fig. 8, three additional steps in the CM-PIR flowchart are included for the biometric authentication classification only. With that, two more feature calculations are made on the CM-PIR data for concatenation to be utilized in the biometric authentication classification of Subject A against all other adversaries.

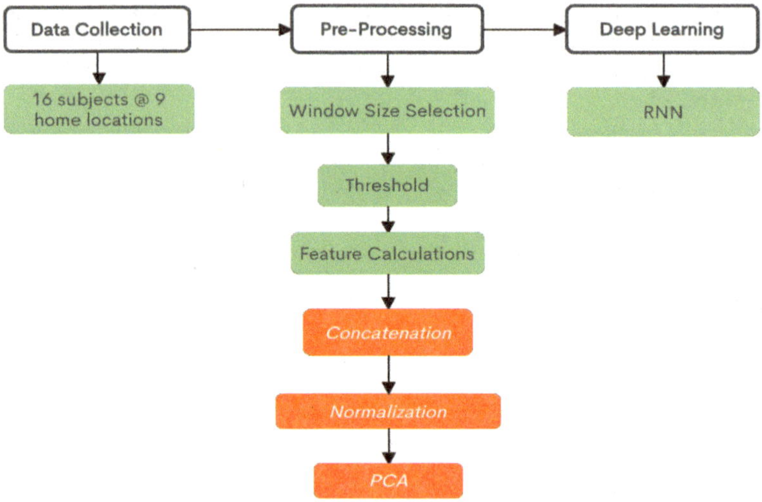

Fig. 8 CM-PIR flow chart. The orange is for biometric authentication only and the green is for both human detection and biometric authentication classifications

The first additional feature to be used for biometric authentication is the acceleration filter that models the response of the heart from the chest motion movement. The absolute value of this feature is computed and concatenated to the signal power value. The last feature to be utilized for the biometric authentication classification is the absolute value of the DWT. The DWT feature allows for the frequency and time in location of the raw PIR data to be represented in one feature and has been utilized in related work for biometric authentication. Thus, the absolute value of the FFT, acceleration filter, and DWT are concatenated for biometric authentication in this work.

For the concatenated feature set to be of relative magnitude, we applied the sklearn min max normalization to map the values from zero to one. Following this normalization, PCA was then applied to reduce the dimensionality of the feature set from 2700 data points to five data points. Not only does PCA reduce the dimensionality of the normalized, concatenated feature set, but it also works to identify the values that are representative of the entire vector. As such, PCA increased the accuracy of the biometric authentication classification. Once PCA was applied, the 900-sample human detection feature set and the feature set of five for biometric authentication could be applied to the RNN DL model.

4.3 Recurrent Neural Network (RNN)

To learn the complex feature set originating from the chest motion data captured by one analog PIR sensor, a DL model is proposed. In that case, a similar RNN model to that of the MI-PIR classifications is developed. A similar RNN is proposed in this case due to the success that the RNN shown in classifying time-series data from the MI-PIR system. Towards this, the RNN consists of two LSTM layers, three dropout layers, and two dense layers. The LSTM layers are composed of 128 dimensions and the dense layers are composed of 16 dimensions. The dropout layers have a weight of 0.1 to aid in overfitting, which was initially a problem with a relatively limited dataset for biometric authentication. All the layers of the RNN model utilize the ReLu activation function except for the last dense layer which utilizes the softmax activation function. In terms of the loss function and optimizer utilized in this model, the sparse categorical crossentropy loss function and Adam optimizer are again utilized. Both classifications underwent 125 epochs. We direct the reader to our previous work for a visual representation of the RNN architecture used with CM-PIR [14] The results of these classifications will be presented in the subsequent sub-sections.

4.4 *Human Detection*

The human detection classification achieved 94% accuracy after training on 291 samples and testing on 63 samples as a resultant of a 70% training, 15% testing, 15% validation split. In comparison to the MI-PIR system, CM-PIR achieved lower detection accuracy using one analog PIR sensor; however, the CM-PIR system requires less additional architecture. Utilizing only the analog PIR sensor and the microcontroller for data transmission, the set-up time and cost is much lower with CM-PIR. In comparison to other proposed models for stationary human presence detection using one PIR sensor, the CM-PIR system utilizes less additional hardware. As a standalone PIR sensor that relies on software processing and statistical learning for accurate classification, the novel CM-PIR system advances the capabilities of PIR sensor human monitoring. Based on the chest motion data at a 1-m distance, the CM-PIR system would accurately respond to a desk situation in which the human subject was completely motionless.

4.5 *Biometric Authentication*

The biometric authentication system based on the chest motion data captured by a PIR sensor achieved an accuracy of 75%. These initial results prove the potential efficacy of using a PIR sensor for security purposes. With pre-processed data collection of 12 individuals at six different home locations, the PIR sensor had to differentiate the many ambient environments from the human subjects, as well as authenticate the users based on their unique chest motion movement. With less ambient environments collected for in the data collection process, we hypothesize that these initial results would increase, as with related non-contact biometric authentication systems, data collection occurred at only one central location. In terms of PIR sensors, multiple testing locations causes even more ambient interference in recording of chest motion data. The CM-PIR recorded accuracy, however, is much more robust as a biometric authentication system due to the many ambient environments. As with many systems that rely on DL for classification, we hypothesize that increased data collection of the subjects involved in the study would increase the accuracy of the results. Due to the balancing of an optimal window size selection in terms of data points and data samples, there are limited 90 s batches to learn from. Increasing the data collection efforts could improve the results, especially in the cases of those subjects that were completely removed from the study due to the applied threshold.

4.6 Quantification

New in this work is the addition of the quantification of the maximum sensing distance of the CM-PIR system for accurate detection of stationary human subjects. As the original data collection was present at a 1-m distance, we extend the CM-PIR system for possible detection at a 2 m and 3 m distance. In this quantification, data was collected by Subject A at Location D for 30 min at 1 m, 2 m, and 3 m, with an additional equal time length of unoccupied data collection. In a similar methodology of removing the dataset of longest distance iteratively from the DL model, 3 m was classified with 85% accuracy and 2 m was classified with 92% accuracy. At 1 m, with one ambient environment and one subject, the CM-PIR system detected human subjects with 96% accuracy. With these results in mind, a 1-m distance is proven to be the maximum sensing distance for an accurate stationary human detection system.

5 Discussion

PIR sensors are discussed as potential long-term monitoring solutions due to their low cost, non-contact, non-intrusive, and relatively accurate and reliable results. In terms of cost, the Panasonic AMN 24112 PIR sensor used in both systems proposed in this work costs roughly $30 USD, whereas the Microsoft Kinect sensor used in video-based solutions costs roughly $75 USD. This comparison in cost can be illuminated further when systems rely on multiple video-based modalities for accurate detection, and whereas the proposed solutions in this work require only one sensor modality [54]. Furthermore, the Impinj RAIN RFID reader that is used in related work can cost upwards of $1000 USD [38]. From this, one can identify that the proposed PIR sensor-based systems for human detection and biometric authentication are relatively inexpensive in comparison to systems proposed in related work due to their reliance on only a single COTS sensor modality. With

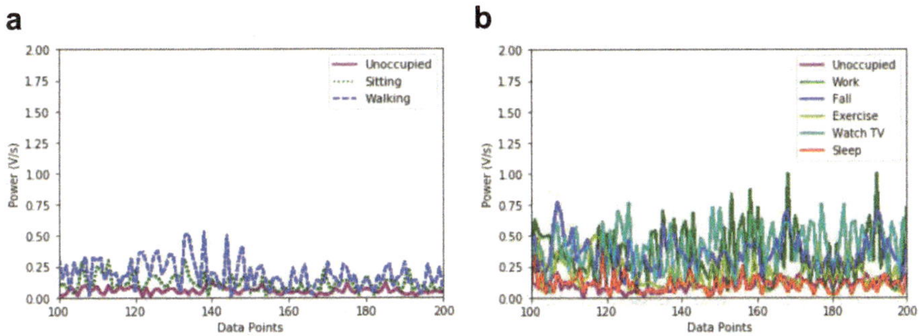

Fig. 9 FFT plot of HAR in (**a**) an office environment and (**b**) a residential environment indicating the differences seen between activities

that, the non-contact, non-intrusive, and accurate nature of PIR sensors makes them suitable modalities for long-term monitoring systems.

The major known drawback with PIR sensors is their inability to detect stationary human subjects reliably and accurately in their FoV. In this work we have introduced two novel systems to combat this major known issue with PIR sensors. MI-PIR is a motion induced PIR sensor system that classifies an office space for room occupancy, occupancy count, relative and precise location, human target differentiation, and simple HAR every 36 s of rotation time. In a residential environment, MI-PIR classified relative and precise locations of one individual subject, as well as showed the efficacy of a more complex HAR classification. CM-PIR on the other hand deploys one PIR sensor in the traditional sense for accurate human detection and biometric authentication for security of IoT devices.

The signal power, or the absolute value of the computed FFT coefficients from the raw PIR voltage data, proved to be a strong feature for the detection of stationary human subjects using an analog PIR sensor. To alleviate the black-box stigma that surrounds DL classification models, we present Fig. 9 which identifies one 36 s batch of each activity collected for during the MI-PIR office and residential data collection. Figure 9(a) indicates the varying signal power for each activity completed in the office environment and Fig. 9(b) indicates the varying signal power for each activity completed in the residential environment. The office environment presents the walking situation to have a greater signal power than the sitting situation, with the unoccupied scenario showing significantly lower signal power. The residential environment signal power comparison presents varying signals that align with our hypotheses. During a work scenario in which the user is seated, working, and using electronics, there would be higher levels of signal power than during the sleep and unoccupied data collections. In a direct comparison of two activities at the same location, "Watching TV on Bed" and "Sleeping on Bed", the latter activity had much less signal power due to both the lack of electronics in use, as well as the lack of movement while sleeping.

Table 6 Comparison of novel systems for stationary human presence detection using one PIR sensor. The models are compared for their solution, methods, FoV, maximum sensing distance, and stationary human presence detection accuracy

Classification	Reference	Proposed solution	Methods	Horizontal FoV (°)	Max. sensing (m)	Accuracy (%)
Stationary human presence	Juan et al. [18]	Optical shutter	Presence—Voltage	110	7	100
	Wu and Wang [22]	Optical shutter	Presence—Voltage	93	4.5	100
	MI-PIR	Motion induced	Classification—RNN	223	19	100
	CM-PIR	Chest motion	Presence—RNN	93	1	94

For comparison of these proposed systems to systems of related work, we highlight Table 6 which includes this information. MI-PIR, CM-PIR, and related work on using a PIR sensor for stationary human presence detection is compared in this Table. MI-PIR through rotation of the analog PIR sensor extends the manufacturer reported horizontal FoV from 93 to 223° through a 130° rotation. In addition, based off the maximum sensing distance quantification, the maximum sensing distance of a stationary human subject was found to be 21 m. For CM-PIR, these results are the manufacturer stated 93° through the deployment in a traditional sense and a 1 m maximum sensing distance. In comparison to related work, MI-PIR extends the FoV for monitoring and extends the maximum sensing distance. For CM-PIR, the FoV, maximum sensing distance, and accuracy is reduced. CM-PIR is however the only solution that requires no additional hardware. As MI-PIR is less mechanically complex than the other systems in related work that require the development of an optical shutter for the analog PIR sensor, CM-PIR requires no robotic actuator for accurate stationary human presence detection.

In terms of differentiating the results of the MI-PIR system with related work in HAR classification, the MI-PIR proves superior as presented in Table 7. MI-PIR produces a higher accuracy of differentiating unoccupied, sitting, and walking activities than in related work. From a 100% accuracy to a 93% accuracy, one can determine that the MI-PIR system is more accurate as a simple HAR classification. Although classification in the related work is through a continuous data collection with multiple people, the accuracy of the MI-PIR system with multiple activities in a residential environment ensures the potential superior efficacy to the related work [22]. The MI-PIR system for classification of a residential environment is compared to the results of the *ALPAS* system presented earlier. This system requires two PIR sensors for HAR classification, whereas the MI-PIR system requires only one analog PIR sensor. The accuracy of the MI-PIR system of classifying five activities with one unoccupied scenario achieves a significantly higher accuracy than the reported F-measure of the *ALPAS* system. Although the ALPAS system classifies four activities at one location with multiple users participating in the study, the MI-PIR system's significant increase in accuracy ensures the superior efficacy to the *ALPAS* system [48].

For comparison of CM-PIR with other biometric authentication systems, CM-PIR classifies one human subject against 11 other individuals that remain in the study following an applied threshold. The 75% accuracy of CM-PIR is compared against the introduced *Cardiac Scan* system of 98.6% accuracy with 78 different subjects. Although the *Cardiac Scan* system achieves much greater accuracy, there are a variety of differences between the two systems that highlights the potential positives that CM-PIR might provide. CM-PIR collects data from nine different ambient environments, although three of which are removed with a threshold during pre-processing. In contrast, *Cardiac Scan* collects data at one central location. The multiple ambient environments that the CM-PIR system must learn from is hypothesized to decrease the accuracy and will be tested in future work. The PIR sensor in which CM-PIR relies on is a passive sensor, and *Cardiac Scan* utilizes an

Table 7 HAR and biometric authentication classification accuracy comparison against similar proposed systems in literature

Classification	Reference	# of PIRs	# of activities	Activities	Results
HAR—Office	Wu and Wang [22]	1	3	– Unoccupied – Sitting – Walking	93% accuracy
	MI-PIR	1	3	– Unoccupied – Sitting – Walking	100% accuracy
HAR—Residential	Kashimoto et al. [48]	2	4	– Eat on sofa – Read of sofa – Use phone on sofa – Use PC on sofa	57% F-measure
	MI-PIR	1	6	– Unoccupied – Working at desk – Laying on ground – Exercise on ground – Watch TV on bed – Sleep on bed	98% accuracy

active Doppler Scanner for biometric authentication [66]. The passive nature of the sensor would allow for greater state-of-mind with less chance of any adverse health and energy concerns.

6 Conclusions

Elderly monitoring remains an ever-growing challenge due to the increasing number of individuals and the prevalence of neurodegenerative diseases found in this population. Current systems for monitoring aging subjects often rely on camera-based or terminal-based modalities that cause both a privacy intrusion and burden to the end-user. Ambient sensors have been proposed to fill the gaps towards a need for non-contact and non-intrusive monitoring systems that provide both accurate localization and HAR classification of aging individuals in a residential environment. Many of these current systems require expensive architecture or multiple sensors deployed throughout the room to expand the FoV. Towards the goal of accurate localization, HAR, and other occupancy related parameters, a novel system coined MI-PIR was proposed in this work. CM-PIR is proposed in this work for human detection and biometric authentication. To summarize the contributions of these two systems, the accuracies and quantifications are included below.

In summary, MI-PIR has shown these results in an office environment utilizing statistical learning . . .

- 100% accurate at room classification,
- 93% accurate at occupancy count estimation,
- 95% accurate at relative location classification,
- 94% accurate at human target differentiation,
- 100% accurate at simple HAR,
- 493.7 cm^2 MSE was quantified for precise indoor localization with varying subject conditions,
- 426.4 cm^2 MSE was quantified for precise indoor localization of Subject 1 only.

MI-PIR has also shown accurate results in a residential environment utilizing statistical learning . . .

- 98% accuracy at relative location classification,
- 98% accurate at differentiating five activities and an unoccupied scenario.
- 131.4 cm^2 was quantified for precise indoor localization of Subject 1 only.

CM-PIR has shown to be accurate in two different classifications . . .

- 94% accurate at human detection of perfectly stationary human subjects,
- 75% accurate at biometric authentication of 13 labels at six varying environments.

These results highlight the potential success of MI-PIR as a long-term elderly monitoring solution and CM-PIR as both a monitoring solution and biometric authentication modality. In the case of HAR for MI-PIR, similar results to those reported above can be obtained via the monitoring of one elderly subject, whereas additional tests are required to determine the efficacy of HAR with many individuals present in an indoor environment. For each other classification, multiple subjects were included, and the results can be directly mapped to a real-world scenario. The only requirement for deployment of MI-PIR would be to collect initial training data of the ambient environment.

While MI-PIR is proposed as a potential elderly monitoring system, CM-PIR is proposed as a combined office space occupancy detection and IoT security system. The FoV of the CM-PIR system is constrained to the manufacturer stated FoV, as this analog PIR sensor is deployed in the traditional sense. As such, CM-PIR is proposed to be deployed at the desk location of a human subject present in an office scenario. Accurate detection of a human subject, even in the most motionless of instances, would aid in smart energy management applications in an office environment. The novelty of the CM-PIR system for stationary human presence detection against proposed methods, including MI-PIR, is the lack of additional hardware and set-up needed. In comparison to a state-of-the-art non-contact biometric authentication system, CM-PIR proves less accurate, but proposes a more adequate sensor modality for long-term monitoring. Data collection at one central location, as well as a greater data collection effort, is hypothesized to increase the initial results of CM-PIR for biometric authentication. CM-PIR would be suitable for human detection in a real-world office environment, but only suitable as a biometric authenticator in a closed room with a single individual. The CM-PIR biometric authentication system extends the capabilities of biometric authentication systems from traditional contact systems to an additional non-contact system. Non-contact and non-intrusive biometric authentication systems for IoT security is a growing need with the ever-growing field of IoT devices in our everyday life.

The summarized results also indicate the efficacy of the RNN model at classifying various scenarios. The RNN proved the most accurate DL model, indicating the temporal reliance of the signal power feature calculated in data pre-processing. With precise indoor localization using a GPR model, MI-PIR showed to be effective at visually clustering locations in two ambient environments, allowing for regression of future coordinate systems during real-world deployment of the system. These activities differentiated in the residential environment proved the potential success as an elderly monitoring modality. In fact, classifying a "Laying on Ground" activity proved direct translation to a potential fall event. Accurately classifying multiple activities that are performed at the same location proves the HAR classification accuracy is not based on the learning of the location in which the activity is performed.

The future of monitoring is in the deployment of ambient sensors with statistical learning algorithms for accurate localization and HAR classification. To fulfill the needs of a non-contact, non-intrusive, low-cost, and passive sensor modality for monitoring situations, a PIR sensor is proposed and highlighted in this work. Solving the known drawback of PIR sensors in this work with two novel systems, the capabilities of PIR sensors for monitoring have been extended. Future work for progression of these two novel systems include testing the MI-PIR system for a real-world data collection and increasing the biometric authentication accuracy of the CM-PIR system. A more systematic data collection and increased data collection is proposed to increase the biometric authentication accuracy of the CM-PIR system. These novel systems highlight the growing field of ambient sensing for human detection and biometric authentication.

Acknowledgments This research is supported by AFOSR grant FA9550-18-1-0287.

References

1. United Nations, D. of E. and S. A. P. D. (2020). *World population ageing 2019* (ST/ESA/SER.A/444). Retrieved from https://www.un.org/development/desa/pd/sites/www.un.org.development.desa.pd/files/files/documents/2020/Jan/un_2019_worldpopulationageing_report.pdf.
2. Milken Institute School of Public Health at The George Washington University. (2018, April 6). *The growing cost of aging in America Part 1: An aging population and rising health care costs*. Retrieved from https://onlinepublichealth.gwu.edu/resources/cost-of-aging-healthcare/.
3. Vespa, J., Armstrong, D. M., & Medina, L. (2020, February). *Demographic turning points for the United States: Population projections for 2020 to 2060*. United States Census Bureau. Retrieved from https://www.census.gov/library/publications/2020/demo/p25-1144.html.
4. de Nardi, M., French, E., Jones, J. B., & McCauley, J. (2015, June). *Medical spending of the elderly*. National Bureau of Economic Research. Retrieved from https://www.nber.org/bah/2015no2/medical-spending-elderly#:~:text=Medical%20spending%20by%20the%20elderly,percent%20of%20all%20medical%20spending.
5. Gitler, A. D., Dhillon, P., & Shorter, J. (2017). Neurodegenerative disease: Models, mechanisms, and a new hope. *Disease Models & Mechanisms, 10*(5). https://doi.org/10.1242/dmm.030205.
6. Gómez-Gómez, M. E., & Zapico, S. C. (2019). Frailty, cognitive decline, neurodegenerative diseases and nutrition interventions. *International Journal of Molecular Sciences, 20*(11). https://doi.org/10.3390/ijms20112842.
7. Agrawal, M., & Biswas, A. (2015). Molecular diagnostics of neurodegenerative disorders. *Frontiers in Molecular Biosciences, 2*. https://doi.org/10.3389/fmolb.2015.00054.
8. Obaidat, M. S., Rana, S. P., Maitra, T., Giri, D., & Dutta, S. (2019). Biometric security and internet of things (IoT). In M. S. Obaidat, I. Traore, & I. Woungang (Eds.), *Biometric-based physical and cybersecurity systems* (pp. 477–509). Springer International Publishing. https://doi.org/10.1007/978-3-319-98734-7_19
9. Alraja, M. N., Farooque, M. M. J., & Khashab, B. (2019). The effect of security, privacy, familiarity, and trust on users' attitudes toward the use of the IOT-based healthcare: The mediation role of risk perception. *IEEE Access, 7*. https://doi.org/10.1109/ACCESS.2019.2904006.
10. Adjabi, I., Ouahabi, A., Benzaoui, A., & Taleb-Ahmed, A. (2020). Past, present, and future of face recognition: A review. *Electronics, 9*(8). doi:https://doi.org/10.3390/electronics9081188.
11. Adra, B. (2019). Facing the facts on biometric phone locks: Your face and thumb are not secure.
12. Yang, W., Hu, J., Wang, S., & Wu, Q. (2018). Biometrics based privacy-preserving authentication and mobile template protection. *Wireless Communications and Mobile Computing, 2018*. https://doi.org/10.1155/2018/7107295.
13. Andrews, J., Kowsika, M., Vakil, A., & Li, J. (2020a). A motion induced passive infrared (PIR) sensor for stationary human occupancy detection. In *2020 IEEE/ION position, location and navigation symposium (PLANS)*, pp. 1295–1304.
14. Andrews, J., Vakil, A., & Li, J. (2020b, December 5). Biometric authentication and stationary detection of human subjects by deep learning of passive infrared (PIR) sensor data. In *IEEE signal processing in medicine and biology (SPMB) 2020*.

15. Hobbie, R. K., & Roth, B. J. (2015). Intermediate physics for medicine and biology. In *Intermediate physics for medicine and biology* (5th ed.). Springer International Publishing. https://doi.org/10.1007/978-3-319-12682-1
16. Liu, X., Yang, T., Tang, S., Guo, P., & Niu, J. (2020b, April 16). From relative azimuth to absolute location. In *Proceedings of the 26th annual international conference on mobile computing and networking*. https://doi.org/10.1145/3372224.3380878.
17. Mukhopadhyay, B., Srirangarajan, S., & Kar, S. (2018). Modeling the analog response of passive infrared sensor. *Sensors and Actuators A: Physical, 279*. https://doi.org/10.1016/j.sna.2018.05.002.
18. Juan, R. O. S., Kim, J. S., Sa, Y. H., Kim, H. S., & Cha, H. W. (2016). Development of a sensing module for standing and moving human body using a shutter and PIR sensor. *International Journal of Multimedia and Ubiquitous Engineering, 11*(7). https://doi.org/10.14257/ijmue.2016.11.7.05.
19. University Recieves $1 Milllion for Transformational Energy Technology. (2018, January 23). *Stony brook matters: News for Alumni & Friends*. Retrieved from https://news.stonybrook.edu/stony-brook-matters/alumni/university-receives-1-million-for-transformational-energy-technology/
20. Wang, Y. (2020). *Current research projects*. Nanomaterial Energy Harvesting and Sensing (NES) Lab. Retrieved from https://yawang08.wixsite.com/yawang/blank-c151z.
21. Wu, L., Gou, F., Wu, S.-T., & Wang, Y. (2020). SLEEPIR: Synchronized low-energy electronically chopped PIR sensor for true presence detection. *IEEE Sensors Letters, 4*(3). https://doi.org/10.1109/LSENS.2020.2976801.
22. Wu, L., & Wang, Y. (2019). A low-power electric-mechanical driving approach for true occupancy detection using a shuttered passive infrared sensor. *IEEE Sensors Journal, 19*(1). https://doi.org/10.1109/JSEN.2018.2875659.
23. Wu, L., & Wang, Y. (2020, September 15). True presence detection via passive infrared sensor network using liquid crystal infrared shutters. In *ASME 2020 conference on smart materials, adaptive structures and intelligent systems*. https://doi.org/10.1115/SMASIS2020-2366.
24. Wu, L., Wang, Y., & Liu, H. (2018). Occupancy detection and localization by monitoring nonlinear energy flow of a shuttered passive infrared sensor. *IEEE Sensors Journal, 18*(21). https://doi.org/10.1109/JSEN.2018.2869555.
25. Shubhendu S., & Vijay, J. (2013). Applicability of artificial intelligence in different fields of life. *International Journal of Scientific Engineering and Research (IJSER), 1*(1).
26. Topol, E. (2019). *Deep medicine*. Basic Books.
27. Hong, X., Gao, J., Jiang, X., & Harris, C. J. (2014). Estimation of Gaussian process regression model using probability distance measures. *Systems Science & Control Engineering, 2*(1). https://doi.org/10.1080/21642583.2014.970731.
28. Zhang, G., Wang, P., Chen, H., & Zhang, L. (2019a). Wireless indoor localization using convolutional neural network and gaussian process regression. *Sensors, 19*(11). https://doi.org/10.3390/s19112508.
29. Abiodun, O. I., Jantan, A., Omolara, A. E., Dada, K. V., Mohamed, N. A., & Arshad, H. (2018). State-of-the-art in artificial neural network applications: A survey. *Heliyon, 4*(11). https://doi.org/10.1016/j.heliyon.2018.e00938.
30. Shrestha, A., & Mahmood, A. (2019). Review of deep learning algorithms and architectures. *IEEE Access, 7*. https://doi.org/10.1109/ACCESS.2019.2912200.
31. Hochreiter, S. (1998). The Vanishing gradient problem during learning recurrent neural nets and problem solutions. *International Journal of Uncertainty, Fuzziness and Knowledge-Based Systems, 6*(2). https://doi.org/10.1142/S0218488598000094.
32. Adadi, A., & Berrada, M. (2018). Peeking inside the black-box: A survey on explainable artificial intelligence (XAI). *IEEE Access, 6*. https://doi.org/10.1109/ACCESS.2018.2870052.
33. Vakil, A. (2020). Heterogenous multimodal sensor fusion via canonical correlation analysis and explainable AI.

34. Li, D., Liu, J., Nishimura, S., Hayashi, Y., Suzuki, J., & Gong, Y. (2020a, October 12). Multi-person action recognition in microwave sensors. In *Proceedings of the 28th ACM international conference on multimedia*. https://doi.org/10.1145/3394171.3413801.
35. Singh, S., & Aksanli, B. (2019). Non-intrusive presence detection and position tracking for multiple people using low-resolution thermal sensors. *Journal of Sensor and Actuator Networks, 8*(3). https://doi.org/10.3390/jsan8030040.
36. Bianco, V., Mazzeo, P. L., Paturzo, M., Distante, C., & Ferraro, P. (2020). Deep learning assisted portable IR active imaging sensor spots and identifies live humans through fire. *Optics and Lasers in Engineering, 124*. doi:https://doi.org/10.1016/j.optlaseng.2019.105818.
37. Kim, S., Kang, S., Ryu, K. R., & Song, G. (2019). Real-time occupancy prediction in a large exhibition hall using deep learning approach. *Energy and Buildings, 199*. https://doi.org/10.1016/j.enbuild.2019.06.043.
38. Oguntala, G. A., Abd-Alhameed, R. A., Ali, N. T., Hu, Y.-F., Noras, J. M., Eya, N. N., Elfergani, I., & Rodriguez, J. (2019). SmartWall: Novel RFID-enabled ambient human activity recognition using machine learning for unobtrusive health monitoring. *IEEE Access, 7*. https://doi.org/10.1109/ACCESS.2019.2917125.
39. Liu, J., Mu, H., Vakil, A., Ewing, R., Shen, X., Blasch, E., & Li, J. (2020a). Human occupancy detection via passive cognitive radio. *Sensors, 20*(15). https://doi.org/10.3390/s20154248.
40. Fan, L., Li, T., Fang, R., Hristov, R., Yuan, Y., & Katabi, D. (2020a, June). Learning longterm representations for person re-identification using radio signals. In *2020 IEEE/CVF conference on computer vision and pattern recognition (CVPR)*. https://doi.org/10.1109/CVPR42600.2020.01071.
41. Fan, L., Li, T., Yuan, Y., & Katabi, D. (2020b, August). In-home daily-life captioning using radio signals. In *European conference on computer vision (EECV 2020)*.
42. Li, T., Fan, L., Zhao, M., Liu, Y., & Katabi, D. (2019, October). Making the invisible visible: Action recognition through walls and occlusions. In *2019 IEEE/CVF international conference on computer vision (ICCV)*. https://doi.org/10.1109/ICCV.2019.00096.
43. Singh, A. D., Sandha, S. S., Garcia, L., & Srivastava, M. (2019). RadHAR. In *Proceedings of the 3rd ACM workshop on millimeter-wave networks and sensing systems—MmNets'19*. https://doi.org/10.1145/3349624.3356768.
44. Zou, H., Zhou, Y., Yang, J., & Spanos, C. J. (2018). Towards occupant activity driven smart buildings via WiFi-enabled IoT devices and deep learning. *Energy and Buildings, 177*. https://doi.org/10.1016/j.enbuild.2018.08.010.
45. Das, A., Sangogboye, F. C., Raun, E. S. K. & Kjærgaard, M. B. HeteroSense: An Occupancy Sensing Framework for Multi-Class Classification for Activity Recognition and Trajectory Detection. in Proceedings of the Fourth International Workshop on Social Sensing-SocialSense'19 (ACM Press, 2019). https://doi:10.1145/3313294.3313383.
46. Pham, M., Yang, D., & Sheng, W. (2019). A sensor fusion approach to indoor human localization based on environmental and wearable sensors. *IEEE Transactions on Automation Science and Engineering, 16*(1). https://doi.org/10.1109/TASE.2018.2874487.
47. Gochoo, M., Tan, T.-H., Velusamy, V., Liu, S.-H., Bayanduuren, D., & Huang, S.-C. (2017). Device-free non-privacy invasive classification of elderly travel patterns in a smart house using PIR sensors and DCNN. *IEEE Sensors Journal*.https://doi.org/10.1109/JSEN.2017.2771287.
48. Kashimoto, Y., Fujiwara, M., Fujimoto, M., Suwa, H., Arakawa, Y., & Yasumoto, K. (2017, March). ALPAS: Analog-PIR-sensor-based activity recognition system in smarthome. In *2017 IEEE 31st international conference on advanced information networking and applications (AINA)*. https://doi.org/10.1109/AINA.2017.33.
49. Wang, X., Wang, X., Mao, S., Zhang, J., Periaswamy, S. C. G., & Patton, J. (2020). Indoor radio map construction and localization with deep gaussian processes. *IEEE Internet of Things Journal, 7*(11). doi:https://doi.org/10.1109/JIOT.2020.2996564.
50. Zhang, G., Wang, P., Chen, H., & Zhang, L. (2019b). Wireless indoor localization using convolutional neural network and gaussian process regression. *Sensors, 19*(11). https://doi.org/10.3390/s19112508.

51. Zhang, B., Li, S., Huang, Z., Rahi, B. H., Wang, Q., & Li, M. (2018). Transfer learning-based online multiperson tracking with Gaussian process regression. *Concurrency and Computation: Practice and Experience, 30*(23). https://doi.org/10.1002/cpe.4917.
52. He, X., Aloi, D., & Li, J. (2016, January). Portable 3D visual sensor based indoor localization on mobile device. In *2016 13th IEEE annual consumer communications & networking conference (CCNC)*. https://doi.org/10.1109/CCNC.2016.7444947.
53. Burns, E., & Kakara, R. (2018). Deaths from falls among persons aged ≥65 years—United States, 2007–2016. MMWR. *Morbidity and Mortality Weekly Report, 67*(18). https://doi.org/10.15585/mmwr.mm6718a1.
54. Huang, Z., Liu, Y., Fang, Y., & Horn, B. K. P. (2018, October). Video-based fall detection for seniors with human pose estimation. In *2018 4th international conference on Universal Village (UV)*. https://doi.org/10.1109/UV.2018.8642130.
55. Kabelac, Z., Tarolli, C. G., Snyder, C., Feldman, B., Glidden, A., Hsu, C.-Y., Hristov, R., Dorsey, E. R., & Katabi, D. (2019). Passive monitoring at home: A pilot study in Parkinson disease. *Digital Biomarkers, 3*(1). https://doi.org/10.1159/000498922.
56. Vhaduri, S., & Poellabauer, C. (2019). Multi-modal biometric-based implicit authentication of wearable device users. *IEEE Transactions on Information Forensics and Security, 14*(12). https://doi.org/10.1109/TIFS.2019.2911170.
57. Hom Choudhury, S., Kumar, A., & Laskar, S. H. (2019). Biometric authentication through unification of finger dorsal biometric traits. *Information Sciences, 497*. https://doi.org/10.1016/j.ins.2019.05.045.
58. Clark, J. W., Neuman, M. R., Olson, W. H., Peura, R. A., Primiano, F. P., Siedband, M. P., Webster, J. G., & Wheeler, L. A. (2009). In J. G. Webster (Ed.), *Medical instrumentation: Application and design* (4th ed.). Wiley.
59. Zhang, Q. (2018, November). Deep learning of electrocardiography dynamics for biometric human identification in era of IoT. In *2018 9th IEEE annual ubiquitous computing, electronics & mobile communication conference (UEMCON)*. https://doi.org/10.1109/UEMCON.2018.8796676.
60. Wang, D., Si, Y., Yang, W., Zhang, G., & Liu, T. (2019). A novel heart rate robust method for short-term electrocardiogram biometric identification. *Applied Sciences, 9*(1). https://doi.org/10.3390/app9010201.
61. Li, Y., Pang, Y., Wang, K., & Li, X. (2020b). Toward improving ECG biometric identification using cascaded convolutional neural networks. *Neurocomputing, 391*. https://doi.org/10.1016/j.neucom.2020.01.019.
62. Xu, X., Liang, Y., He, P., & Yang, J. (2019). Adaptive motion artifact reduction based on empirical wavelet transform and wavelet thresholding for the non-contact ECG monitoring systems. *Sensors, 19*(13). https://doi.org/10.3390/s19132916.
63. Massaroni, C., Lo Presti, D., Formica, D., Silvestri, S., & Schena, E. (2019). Non-contact monitoring of breathing pattern and respiratory rate via RGB signal measurement. *Sensors, 19*(12). https://doi.org/10.3390/s19122758.
64. Li, F., Valero, M., Shahriar, H., Khan, R. A., & Ahamed, S. I. (2021). Wi-COVID: A COVID-19 symptom detection and patient monitoring framework using WiFi. *Smart Health, 19*. https://doi.org/10.1016/j.smhl.2020.100147.
65. Kapu, H., Saraswat, K., Ozturk, Y., & Cetin, A. E. (2017). Resting heart rate estimation using PIR sensors. *Infrared Physics & Technology, 85*. https://doi.org/10.1016/j.infrared.2017.05.010.
66. Lin, F., Song, C., Zhuang, Y., Xu, W., Li, C., & Ren, K. (2017, October 4). Cardiac scan. In *Proceedings of the 23rd annual international conference on mobile computing and networking*. https://doi.org/10.1145/3117811.3117839.

Generalization of Deep Acoustic and NLP Models for Large-Scale Depression Screening

Amir Harati, Tomasz Rutowski, Yang Lu, Piotr Chlebek, Ricardo Oliveira, Elizabeth Shriberg, and David Lin

1 Introduction and Background

1.1 Depression and Screening

Depression is one of the most common mental health disorders worldwide. It is a prevalent, debilitating condition that is often under-diagnosed [1, 2]. In the United States alone, 17.3 million people (7.1% of the U.S. population) have experienced at least one episode of major depressive disorder [3]. 9.3% of primary care visits and 9.4% of emergency department (ED) visits in the U.S. indicate depression as the primary complaint [4]. The economic costs related to depression average approximately $210.5 billion per year, a 21.5% increase since 2005. Medical care received accounts for 50% of the cost, with the other 50% being workplace-related (absenteeism and presenteeism) [5].

Depression screening, coupled with appropriate intervention, is essential for patients to receive the right treatment. Without screening in primary care, only 50% of patients are diagnosed with depression [6]. Two-thirds of patients present with somatic complaints (physical issues) instead of depressive symptoms [7]. For these reasons, screening is a vital first step to improved health outcomes that can result in increased quality of life, decreased mortality, and decreased costs.

Traditional screening tests can be grouped into two categories: depression assessment scales and symptom count instruments [8]. The first category includes, among others, the Beck Depression Inventory (BDI), the Geriatric Depression Scale (GDS), and the Hospital Anxiety and Depression Scale (HADS). The second

A. Harati (✉) · T. Rutowski · Y. Lu · P. Chlebek · R. Oliveira · E. Shriberg · D. Lin
Ellipsis Health Inc., San Francisco, CA, USA
e-mail: amir@ellipsishealth.com; tomek@ellipsishealth.com; yang@ellipsishealth.com; piotr@ellipsishealth.com; ricardo@ellipsishealth.com; liz@ellipsishealth.com; david@ellipsishealth.com

I. Obeid et al. (eds.), *Biomedical Sensing and Analysis*,
https://doi.org/10.1007/978-3-030-99383-2_3

category includes, among others, the Patient Health Questionnaire (PHQ-9), the Primary Care Evaluation of Mental Disorder (PRIME-MD), and the Symptom-Driven Diagnostic System for Primary Care (SDDS-PC). Ease of administration and interpretability are two main factors when deciding which screening tool should be used in clinical practice. The PHQ-9 has been suggested [8] as the screening test of choice for primary care physicians because it measures both depression criteria and severity; moreover, it is relatively easy to administer compared to tests such as Hamilton Rating Scale for Depression (HAM-D), which should be administered by trained interviewers [8].

However, self-report tests such as the PHQ-9 are not scalable, as some patients (e.g., those with language deficiency, the very old, and the very young, among others) require supervision, while others have difficulty completing them due to their literacy level. In addition, due to their standardized nature, self-report tests are not engaging due to a lack of personalization and the inability of the patient to choose to focus upon what matters to them. Digital health technologies can address these insufficiencies and facilitate the screening and monitoring of depression and other behavioral health conditions to aid providers and care teams. Spoken language technology offers potential advantages for this. Speaking is natural and engaging for patients and does not require special equipment. As shown in a line of past work, speech contains acoustic and language cues that can be captured by machine learning models to predict a speaker's behavioral health state; see e.g., Resnik et al. [9], Cummins et al. [10], Williamson et al. [11], Pampouchidou et al. [12], Yang et al. [13], Ringeval et al. [14], and Rutowski et al. [15].

This chapter introduces machine learning techniques applied to acoustic and text modalities of speech signal. It then provides an analysis of the robustness of these models over different factors concerning speaker characteristics such as age, gender, ethnicity, and recording environment, e.g., recording time. This robustness is impressive considering that the prior depression distribution varies with regard to these factors.

1.2 Background on Machine Learning Approach

Feature engineering was an early and dominant approach in the domain of acoustic models for behavioral health prediction [10, 16]. Sample features include voice quality [17], articulation and coordination [18–20], speech rate [20], and spectral [10], prosodic [21] and formant features [18]. Limited specificity [10, 16], non-standard feature measurement [10], and an overall limited amount of data [10] are among the reasons for inconsistent results and disagreement across different studies.

Conversation analysis [22], i.e. analyzing patient language, was the first type of word-based modeling applied to the behavioral health domain. These analyses include investigation of the meanings of words used and their implications for patient psychological state [23–25]. There are many approaches to analyzing different sources of data. Some of these methods include analyzing electronic health records [26, 27], mobile text messages [28], and forums and social media [29].

In recent years, however, end-to-end models have gained popularity. End-to-end models directly map the input signal to target labels. Advances in deep learning have led to improved results in a range of applications including automatic speech recognition (ASR) [30–32], affect, and behavioral health [33–39]. In contrast to the feature engineering paradigm, the deep end-to-end approach focuses on designing a model that can automatically learn features from data. There has been increased research on the application of deep learning methods for the task of depression prediction. For example, in the natural language processing (NLP) domain, the authors of Yang et al. [13], He and Cao [40], and Yates et al. [29] investigated different deep convolutional networks (CNNs). In Ringeval et al. [14], a CNN pretrained over an image classification task was used as a feature extractor.

Although deep end-to-end methods show strong performance in many applications as observed above, they also face challenges. Two major challenges are the need for large amounts of data and the potential of overfitting. One common approach to address some of these problems is to use transfer learning (TL). Transfer learning has been used in emotion [33, 41–43], PTSD [44], depression [14, 45–47], and anxiety [46] prediction problems.

1.3 Modeling and Analysis Approach

The acoustic model described in this chapter uses transfer learning from an ASR source task to learn a useful representation of the speech signal. Application of transfer learning and ASR tasks specifically is not new; for example, Zhao et al. [47] proposed a hierarchical autoencoder with transfer learning from ASR. The acoustic model described in this chapter, however, uses a simpler architecture, is trained using a simpler procedure, and is designed to be lightweight during the inference time, which is an important practical consideration for commercial deployment.

The NLP model was initially based on a language model pretrained on publicly-available data. Further fine tuning was then done using publicly-available depression corpora as well as the proprietary corpus. The model was then further trained for classification and regression objectives. The combination of various data sets and our training recipe enabled this model to achieve excellent performance; this is reported in subsequent sections.

One important contribution to this work for both acoustic and NLP models is the application of a large corpus with nearly 10,000 unique speakers and 1600 hours of labeled speech. These speech recordings were obtained from sessions in which users interacted with a human-computer application and answered questions about their lives. Gold standard labels for machine predictions were based on standard self-report instruments completed by each speaker within each session. This corpus is several orders of magnitudes larger than the shared dataset in the community [14] and allows proper investigation of the effect of transfer learning, effect of training data size, and robustness of acoustic and NLP models relative to various human and environmental factors.

Robustness has been studied by comparing the performance of models while controlling for an independent factor such age, gender, or ethnicity. An earlier version of these results is also published in Lu et al. [48]. Predictions of both acoustic and NLP models are studied for many of these factors and results indicate that the models' performance does not change significantly relative to these factors. Furthermore, experimentation shows that, for the NLP model, performance does not degrade significantly once evaluated on a corpus with different demographics relative to the corpus used for training the model. This result is consistent with conclusions from robustness analysis. It is acknowledged that robustness analysis is only based on data within the same collection (or similar collections), which includes different patients but with similar collection methodology, and therefore, data is considered matched. However, this is a starting point for similar analysis. It is intended that this study will be extended to multiple data collections with different methodologies and demographics.

1.4 Chapter roadmap

The remainder of this chapter is organized as follows. Section two introduces the data sources used in this chapter. Metrics and an overview of modeling approach are also described. Section three describes acoustic models and presents results and experiments using these models. Section four describes NLP models and corresponding results and experimentation. Section five presents an analysis of acoustic and NLP models' robustness. Finally, section six presents a short discussion of this chapter and conclusion.

2 Method

2.1 Data

2.1.1 General Population Corpus

A large set of depression-labeled data from speakers with different backgrounds was needed for model training and evaluation. For this reason, proprietary data was used instead of shared but much smaller corpora [14, 49, 50]. The data used comprises American English spontaneous speech, with users allowed to speak freely [51] in response to questions within a session. Users were paid for their participation and ranged in age from 18 to over 65 years, with a mean age of roughly 30. They interacted with a software application that presented questions on different topics, such as "work" or "Home life". Responses averaged about

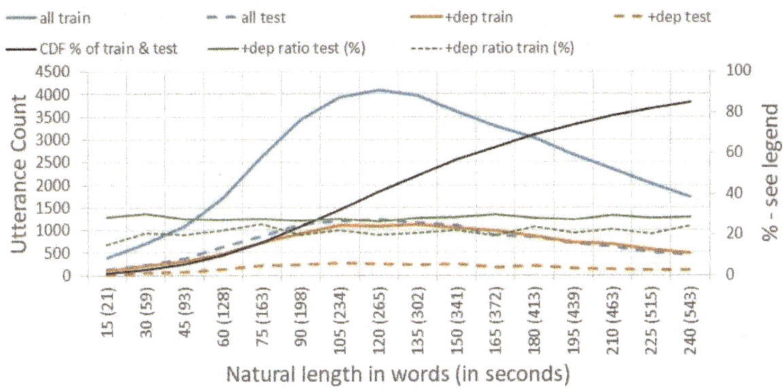

Fig. 1 Distribution of word lengths in the General Population

Table 1 Data characteristics. Number of sessions and speakers for dep+, dep−, and total data for General Population (GP) and Senior Population (SP) groups are shown. dep +/− shows number of data points where sessions for same speaker has changed over time from dep+ to dep− or vice versa

	GP		SP	
	Sessions	Speakers	Sessions	Speakers
dep+ (train)	3606	1863	–	–
dep+ (dev)	326	326	–	–
dep+ (test)	327	327	105	32
dep− (train)	8004	4717	–	–
dep− (dev)	1253	1253	–	–
dep− (test)	1172	1172	378	92
dep +/− (total)	2209	526	204	37
Total	14,688	9658	687	161
Responses	**GP sessions**		**SP sessions**	
Length (words)	~800		~450	
Number/session	4.5		6.1	

125 words—longer than some reports of turn lengths in conversation, e.g., in Jiahong et al. [52] (see Fig. 1). Users responded to 4–6 different questions per session (mean 4.52) using natural speech. After providing their speech responses, users filled out eight questions from the PHQ-9 questionnaire (the ninth question, regarding suicide, was removed, making the survey the PHQ-8). The PHQ-8 has been clinically validated in large studies to reflect depression risk severity [53]. The PHQ-8 score served as the machine learning target label for both the session and the responses within it. Scores were mapped to a binary classification task, with scores at or above 10 mapped to depressed (dep+) and scores below 10 to nondepressed (dep−), following Kroenke et al. [53]; see Table 1. Data was partitioned into train, development, and test subsets. The train, development, and test partitions contained no overlapping speakers. Test and development splits were approximately the same size and contained unique speakers; 43% of sessions in the train split were from repeated users. The distribution of PHQ-8 values in our General Population (GP) corpus is shown in Fig. 2.

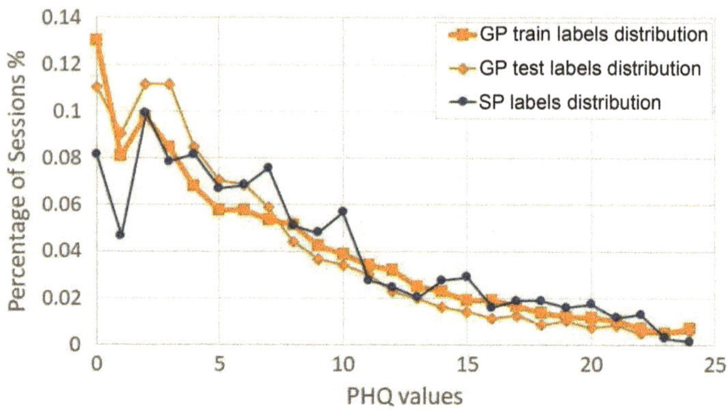

Fig. 2 PHQ distribution

As shown in Fig. 1, data partitions are well-matched, including nearly identical CDFs (black lines overlap) and similar distributions for class lengths both within and across partitions. Depression priors (i.e., dep+) differ slightly, at 28% for train vs. 22% for test data.

The corpus contains metadata including self-reported information about the user and automatically-generated information about session timing. User metadata under consideration in this chapter includes gender, age group, smoking habits, ethnicity, marital status, and location. Table 2 compares the composition of user demographics in the General Population corpus with the US population between the ages of 18–65 [54, 55]. Gender, age, and ethnicity compositions for the train, development, and test sets as well as for the US population are shown. The General Population corpus represents the US population's ethnic and gender composition well, with the corpus having a higher female population than male. In terms of age, the General Population corpus is more reflective of the younger population. It contains more people in the 26–35 category and fewer from the 46–65 category compared to the US population.

Session metadata includes information about session administration, including the following characteristics: local time of day, day of the week, and season during which the session was recorded. In our collection, users were allowed to choose their recording days and times. Interestingly, differences were found in both the frequency of recording and the PHQ-8 value priors. As an example of the latter, even after averaging over more than 16,000 sessions and 10,000 users, sessions that occurred at certain times of day (local to the user's time zone) were more likely to be marked positive for depression (dep+) than sessions collected at other times of day. This pattern varies relatively smoothly, as shown in Fig. 3.

Table 2 General Population speaker demographic comparison with US population

Subset	Sub-category	Total speakers	Train speakers	Test speakers	US population between age 18–65[a]
Total user count[a]		9658	6580	3078	
Gender	Female	58.9%	58.9%	58.7%	50.2%
	Male	40.6%	40.3%	40.8%	49.8%
	Other	0.7%	0.7%	0.5%	N/A
Age[b]	18–25	29.3%	30.0%	28.0%	17.0%
	26–35	43.7%	42.9%	45.7%	22.3%
	36–45	17.4%	17.7%	17.0%	20.1%
	46–65	9.0%	8.8%	9.4%	40.6%
Ethnicity	Caucasian	68.8%	69.4%	67.4%	73.0%
	Hispanic and Latino	7.7%	7.5%	8.2%	17.6%
	Black or African American	7.5%	7.3%	8.0%	12.7%
	More than one race	5.5%	5.4%	5.7%	3.1%
	East Asian	4.0%	4.0%	4.2%	All Asian: 5.4%
	South Asian	2.1%	2.8%	2.0%	
	Other	4.3%	4.3%	4.6%	4.8%

[a] The demographic composition of the GP corpus is compared against the US population of age 18–65 [54, 55]

[b] Percentages in each category may not add up to one due to missing data or users' choice of not sharing that information

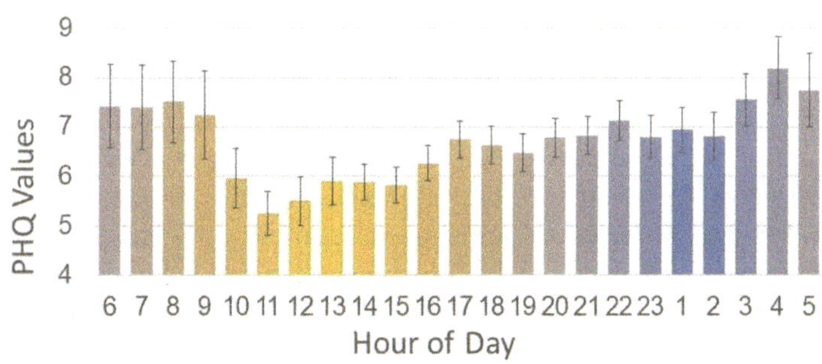

Fig. 3 PHQ-8 values (mean and variance) for sessions by time of day the session was recorded (local time), for full corpus. The colorization loosely corresponds to the time of day (daytime or nighttime)

2.1.2 Senior Population Corpus

A second set of data, the Senior Population (SP) corpus, was collected from a population of older speakers. This corpus was used to further evaluate the generalization of the word-based model. Speech elicitation and incentives for this corpus were similar to those in Sect. 2.1.1 for the General Population corpus, allowing for comparisons to generally focus on the characteristics of the speakers rather than the task. Corpus statistics are given in Table 1.

The Senior Population corpus was collected in Southern California through an Ellipsis Health partner. The partner is associated with a group practice site comprising over 100 primary care doctors and 200 specialists caring for more than 40,000 patients. For both corpora, labels were based on self-reports using the PHQ-8 collected at the end of each session. The demographic breakdown of the population in age and gender is given in Table 3.

A positive (dep+) sample of the General Population is provided below:

> "Right now, I'm living with my husband and my two daughters and I am a stay-at-home mom I lost my job when I was pregnant with my second daughter and honestly it's been a roller coaster expected to be fine at home take care kids but it's the most stressful thing I've ever done and I cannot wait to go back to work."

A positive (dep+) sample of the Senior Population response is provided below:

> "My home life is good and it with my sister we have an amazing relationship and we don't get upset with each other very often and when we do get upset with each other were always able to find a medium a meeting area that we can work together to get beyond it or to just realize that it's okay to sometimes be different have a great home life."

2.1.3 Pretraining Data

To take advantage of the large benefits of transfer learning methods (see Sect. 2.3), additional data sources were obtained for the pretraining stages of the acoustic and NLP tasks. This was also due to the proprietary labelled General Population dataset, which in terms of size is large compared to publicly-available depression datasets but relatively small for the deep learning methods used in this chapter.

Table 3 Senior Population user demographics

Total: 161		
Gender	Male	60.0%
	Female	40.0%
Age	<55	16.9%
	55–59	14.0%
	60–64	11.0%
	65–69	33.8%
	≥70	24.3%

For language model training, additional data was collected. There are many publicly-available websites or forums wherein depressed people talk about themselves. Over a million such utterances were collected to further strengthen the NLP language models; that is, such data was not used for classification purposes but only to enrich the language model itself. In addition, for general NLP language model training, the following two corpora were used. The first is the Wikipedia subset from Merity et al. [56]; additional data also included part of the Schwenk et al. [57] large data corpus.

For the acoustic model pretraining and transfer learning stage, LibriSpeech [58] was used. LibriSpeech is an English read speech dataset that contains over 1000 h of speech. In this chapter, it was used to train an ASR module which was used as one of the stages in the transfer learning process discussed in the following sections.

2.2 *Metrics and Significance Testing*

This section describes the metrics used for measuring the performance of binary classification and regression tasks. For the binary classification task, a threshold of 10 was used (as suggested by Kroenke et al. [53]) to categorize the data into dep+ and dep− classes. The quality of the classifiers was evaluated using a receiver operating characteristic (ROC) curve showing their performances at all classification thresholds. The ROC curve plots sensitivity of a model against its recall, which is (1-specificity), showing the tradeoff of system performance between sensitivity and specificity. The area under the curve (AUC) value was used as a metric of the binary classification model ability to separate dep+ from dep− classes. In general, a good classifier with higher separation power has its curve closer to the left upper corner and an AUC value closer to 1. A random model has no predictive power and the ROC curve is a straight line from the lower-left to the upper-right corner, where the AUC value is 0.5. Specificity and sensitivity were also calculated at the equal error rate (EER) point; the results are reported in subsequent sections.

The performance of the model across different subsets was compared using AUC values and the DeLong test [59] was used to verify statistical significance; $p \leq 0.05$ was used as the cutoff for statistical significance, i.e., to indicate that the model performance in AUC was statistically significantly higher or lower for sessions in the subset compared to its complement. Due to the large size of the dataset, the fast implementation of the DeLong test [60] was used to reduce the computation time from quadratic to linearithmic.

For regression tasks, root mean square error (RMSE), mean absolute error (MAE), and Pearson correlation (PCC) were used. RMSE and MAE have been used by many authors to report the results of regression tasks, e.g., in AVEC competitions [14]. PCC is also used in some studies [61, 62] and indicates how one variable changes in relation to the other.

2.3 Overview of Modeling Approach

Modeling is described in detail in Sects. 3 and 4, but there are some shared aspects which are discussed here. All models discussed in this chapter are implemented using Pytorch [63] and need GPU for training. However, inference can be performed using CPU.

It is commonly known that deep learning networks require large amounts of data. Behavioral health data is often limited in size, number of positive class examples, or both [14]. For these reasons, transfer learning (TL) is often considered a necessary step for most deep learning tasks [64]. Some of the models described in the following sections take advantage of transfer learning in various ways.

In the traditional machine learning scenario, each task requires a separate learning system that is built from scratch. However, a lot of knowledge can be learned from different related or unrelated tasks [65, p. 41]. Examples of such knowledge include structural similarities or linguistic features for NLP models and acoustic representation for acoustic models.

There are two main steps in the transfer learning process. The first step is to train the model from scratch on the source task. The most common source task for NLP models is training a language model; this is done primarily on large, commonly-available text corpora, e.g., web crawl, Wikipedia, etc. For acoustic models, there is no consensus on the choice of source task, so this choice is often related to the availability of data. In this chapter, language modeling is used as the source task for NLP modeling and ASR as the source task for acoustic modeling.

Adaptation or fine tuning is the second main step of the transfer learning process. There are a few methods for fine tuning that can be done individually or in a combined fashion. Adaptation may require architectural changes in the model wherein additional blocks of the network may be added or removed. Another method is to optimize the network, during which e.g., certain network layers may be frozen from training. At the adaptation stage in this study, text or audio was used as an input and PHQ-8 questionnaire scores as an output. For the purpose of depression screening, a regression or classification function was applied.

The following sections describe details of acoustic and NLP models and then emphasize how transfer learning is applied to these models to obtain state-of-the-art results.

3 Acoustic Models

3.1 Method

3.1.1 Acoustic Features

In order to process raw audio signal using different machine learning algorithms, the analog signal should first be converted to a digital signal using an appropriate sampling scheme. Speech is a wideband signal; however, the information content is usually contained within a relatively narrow bandwidth of 8 kHz [66]. This means that for most applications it is enough to use 16 kHz sampling frequency (based on the Nyquist sampling theorem [67]). In this section, a sampling rate of 16 kHz is used.

Theoretically, digital speech signal (i.e. raw signal) can be used as an input to machine learning algorithms; however, processing this raw signal is computationally expensive. The raw signal, therefore, goes through one more step of feature extraction that reduces the amount of data that needs to be processed by machine learning, while preserving important information.

Filter bank features [68] were computed for the acoustic models described in this chapter. Features were computed using a 25 ms analysis window and 10 ms frame rate over a segment length of 25 s or less. Due to GPU memory limitations, it was not possible to include the full duration of a speaker's session at once. Instead, shorter time segments were created from each session. It was found that longer segments perform better than shorter segments, but longer segments also require more memory. After experimenting with this tradeoff, it was found that 25 s provided the best performance on the development set while staying within hardware memory constraints. Longer durations could be explored given higher-capacity hardware resources.

3.1.2 Acoustic Model

Encoder/Decoder architecture has been used successfully in many speech applications such as ASR [31], speaker verification [69], and emotion recognition [70]. In this architecture, the encoder task is to map the input feature space to a usually lower-dimensional space, and the decoder maps the representation from the aforementioned space into predictions such as posterior probability over classes or intensity of the continuous variable (e.g., in regression problems). The modular architecture allows for flexible training procedures and permits more complex models and algorithms.

This chapter describes an architecture inspired by encoder/decoder models used in ASR applications [30, 31, 71]. In the acoustic model, the encoder consists of a VGG [72] network followed by multiple layers of Bidirectional LSTMs [73]. The decoder (predictor) uses a Recurrent CNN (RCNN) [74] model. In order to prevent confusion with the ASR decoder used in the subsequent section, the name "predictor" is used for the decoder network in the acoustic model.

The input to this model is filter bank coefficients over speech segments with maximum length of 25 s, as mentioned in Sect. 3.1.1. The output of this model is the prediction at segment level. In order to make predictions at the session level, another model is needed; this is discussed in Sect. 3.1.4.

An overview of the acoustic model is provided in Fig. 4 (solid arrows). The speech signal is first divided into segments with a maximum length of 25 s. These segments are then passed to the feature extraction module described in Sect. 3.1.1. The resulting features then pass through the encoder and deep prediction network to obtain a prediction for each individual segment. To compute a session-level

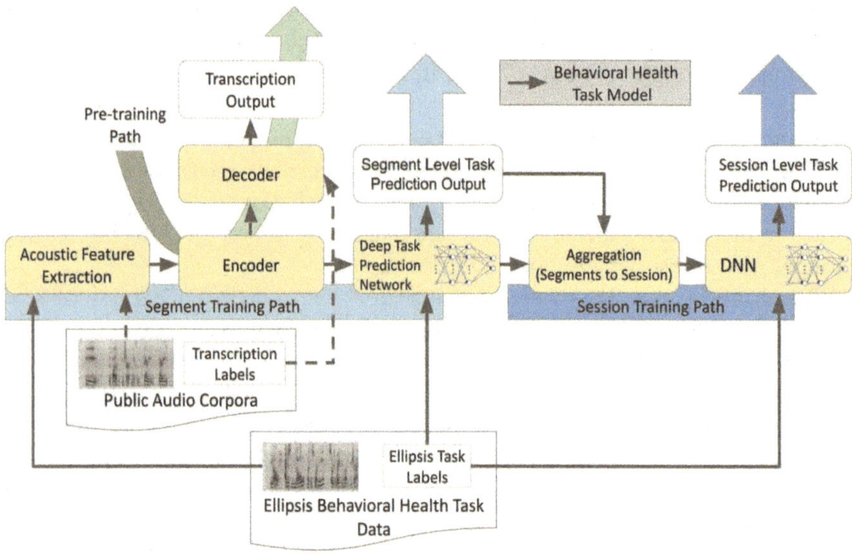

Fig. 4 An overview of the acoustic model. Transfer learning is achieved using an ASR task (dashed arrows). Depression prediction is performed using a pretrained encoder network (solid arrows)

prediction, segment level outputs are aggregated using a segment fusion module, which is discussed in Sect. 3.1.4.

3.1.3 Acoustic with Transfer Learning (Acoustic + TL) Model

Transfer learning is applied to the acoustic model by adding an ASR decoder (hence decoder) module to the network. Results for this model are also published in Harati et al. [75]. The most similar other work that applies transfer learning and deep architecture to the task of predicting depression from speech signal is reported in Zhao et al. [47]. The acoustic + TL model differs from Zhao et al. [47] in its overall architecture, number of modules (acoustic + TL has fewer modules), training steps (acoustic + TL has fewer steps), and transfer learning approach. In Zhao et al. [47], the authors applied both unsupervised and supervised source tasks in their pretraining stage and then transferred the attention weights. In contrast, for the acoustic + TL model, only a supervised task (ASR) is applied, and then only the weights of the encoder are transferred.

In Fig. 4, the transfer learning path is shown with dashed arrows to indicate that it only applies to the pretraining stage. It is removed once the encoder is pretrained. The decoder consists of an LSTM layer with attention. ASR is used as the source task. In the pretraining stage, the encoder and decoder are trained with transcribed speech data (unlabeled for behavioral health). After pretraining, the decoder (dashed arrows) is removed and the rest of the network is trained as mentioned in the previous section using labeled data. The ASR decoder is computationally more expensive than the encoder and predictor modules. The acoustic + TL model is relatively lightweight during inference since the ASR decoder can be removed. This is an important practical advantage during deployment.

The ASR sub-model is based on a hybrid CTC/attention architecture [31] and is inspired by prior work including that in Chan et al. [30], Kim et al. [31] and Liu et al. [71]. The LibriSpeech dataset [58] mentioned in Sect. 2.1.3 was used to train the ASR task. Note that speaking style is unmatched with respect to the General Population data because this data comprises spontaneous speech samples in which users speak freely about their lives. Thus, the ASR model trained on LibriSpeech was not expected to perform well on this data. The goal, rather, was for the model to learn a representation for the acoustic space. Future work is planned for the investigation of corpora in addition to LibriSpeech; this will reveal whether style match is important for the impact of transfer learning in the behavioral health domain.

Past work has shown that transfer learning can improve the performance of machine learning algorithms on new tasks by leveraging data and feature representations learned from other well-studied tasks [33, 64]. It is assumed that by pretraining the encoder, the network is forced to learn a more restrictive representation relative to training all layers from scratch. That is, it is assumed that the first few layers act as an advanced feature extractor for the predictor.

3.1.4 Audio Segment Fusion

The individual segments described in Sects. 3.1.2 and 3.1.3 are fused using an additional neural network. Every segment is represented by a vector corresponding to the last hidden layer of the prediction subnetwork (e.g., RCNN in this case). The sequence of segments for every session is projected into a single vector by max pooling and is then fed into a Multi-Layer Perceptron (MLP) network. The model then can be trained for either classification or regression tasks and the output is interpreted accordingly. The output of this sub-module is a prediction for the overall session.

3.2 Experiments and Results

3.2.1 Results for the General Population Corpus

In this section, results for the acoustic model are presented. The final prediction for each session was computed using the segment fusion module and evaluated using the session PHQ-8 label, either as a binary class (dep+ versus dep−) for classification, or directly as a PHQ-8 value for regression. Results on both

Table 4 Binary classification results for depression prediction. Models with transfer learning are indicated using + TL

Model	AUC	Specificity at EER	Sensitivity at EER
Acoustic + TL-1/dev	0.78	0.70	0.70
Acosutic + TL-1/test	0.79	0.71	0.71
Acoustic + TL-2/dev	0.77	0.71	0.71
Acoustic + TL-2/test	0.79	0.72	0.72
Acoustic/dev	0.62	0.58	0.58
Acoustic/test	0.63	0.59	0.59
CNN/dev	0.60	0.59	0.59
CNN/test	0.60	0.56	0.56
LSTM/dev	0.61	0.59	0.59
LSTM/test	0.58	0.56	0.56

development and test splits are reported. Model parameters were selected using only the development set; the test set was used only for the final evaluation.

Table 4 shows the results of the binary classification task for several models. Specificity and sensitivity are calculated at the ERR point. AUC is reported as the single metric for comparison of different models. The statistical significance of differences in AUC is calculated using the DeLong test as mentioned in Sect. 2.2.

The results of an acoustic model trained from scratch are also shown. Additionally, results using CNN (with six convolutional layers and two fully connected layers) and LSTM (with two LSTM and two fully connected layers) models are included. CNN and LSTM models are among the most-used models and have been applied in earlier studies of depression prediction, including Ringeval et al. [14], Yang et al. [13], He and Cao [40], and Al Hanai et al. [76]. All the models listed perform significantly better than chance (in a DeLong test at $p < 0.05$). CNN, LSTM and the acoustic models all achieve AUC close to 0.60 and a DeLong test shows that the difference among these models is not statistically significant. The acoustic with transfer learning (acoustic + TL) model, however, provides a 27% relative gain over the baseline acoustic model. The DeLong test also shows that adding transfer learning to the acoustic model results in highly significant improvement, with a p-value close to zero.

Two experiments were designed to better understand the effect of transfer learning. In the first experiment (denoted by acoustic + TL-1) an ASR task was trained in the pretraining stage by updating both encoder and decoder weights. This resulted in a relatively "strong" source task. In the second experiment (denoted by acoustic + TL-2), the decoder weights were not updated, resulting in a "weak" source task. The character error rate (CER) was 30% for the first experiment and 188% for the second experiment (due to insertion errors, CER can surpass 100%). Both ASR tasks can be considered weak relative to state-of-the-art ASR models, but clearly one is much weaker than the other. It is evident that, for these models, the gain from transfer learning is virtually the same (not statistically significant under

Table 5 Regression results for depression prediction problem

Model	RMSE	MAE	PCC
Acoustic/dev	5.25	4.11	0.18
Acoustic/test	5.26	4.12	0.21
Acosutic + TL/dev	4.60	3.47	0.51
Acoustic + TL/test	4.70	3.56	0.49

DeLong test); that is, interestingly, most of the gain in performance can be achieved with even a weak ASR task for the pretraining step.

Table 5 shows the performance for the corresponding regression task, i.e. predicting PHQ-8 results directly without class mapping. There is also an improvement for regression results, with a 11% relative reduction for RMSE and 13% relative reduction for MAE. Both binary classification and regression results show remarkably stable performance over development and test sets. This is in contrast to past results using smaller datasets [14, 47], in which performance changes greatly between development and test sets.

3.2.2 Effect of Corpus Size on Transfer Learning

Previous sections introduced the acoustic model and applications of transfer learning for training the model. Results indicate that transfer learning has a significant effect on performance. In this section, the following question is investigated: How is transfer learning gain affected by the amount of labeled training data?

To investigate the role of training dataset size, the full training set is sampled randomly to generate several training subsets. For each sampled subset, a model is trained only on the subset while keeping development and test sets constant. Sampling can be performed on different types of data units. Here, three natural units in the data are investigated: responses, sessions, and speakers. Each speaker has one or more associated sessions. Each session contains multiple responses.

All three sampling approaches (based on responses, sessions, or speakers) result in approximately the same amount of speaking time, but that time is distributed over different numbers of sessions and of speakers. For example, by sampling over speakers, all sessions associated with a selected speaker are maintained. In contrast, by sampling over responses, only some of the responses in a session are preserved. In the case of sampling over responses, the following convention is used: all responses sampled from a given session are collected and then labeled with the label from the original full session. The resulting output sessions are always shorter in duration than the corresponding original sessions. In contrast, for sampling over sessions or over speakers, output sessions are equivalent to the original sessions.

Table 6 shows the amount of speech, number of sessions, and number of speakers for each sampling scheme. For example, the 10%-responses subset contains approximately 114 h of speech data, 9032 sessions, and 5404 speakers (with an average output session length of 45 s). The 10%-sessions subset also contains 114 h of speech but comprises 1165 sessions and 1055 speakers (with an average session

Table 6 Data statistics for different experiments of training data size

Experiment	Amount of speech (h)	Number of sessions	Number of speakers
10%-responses	114	9032	5404
10%-sessions		1165	1055
10%-speakers		1170	660
20%-responses	229	10,877	6249
20%-sessions		2331	1947
20%-speakers		2354	1320
40%-responses	458	11,509	6541
40%-sessions		4663	3363
40%-speakers		4568	2640
60%-responses	690	11,572	6562
60%-sessions		6994	4505
60%-speakers		6985	3960
80%-responses	920	11,603	6578
80%-sessions		9325	5623
80%-speakers		9275	5280
100%	1147	11,610	6580

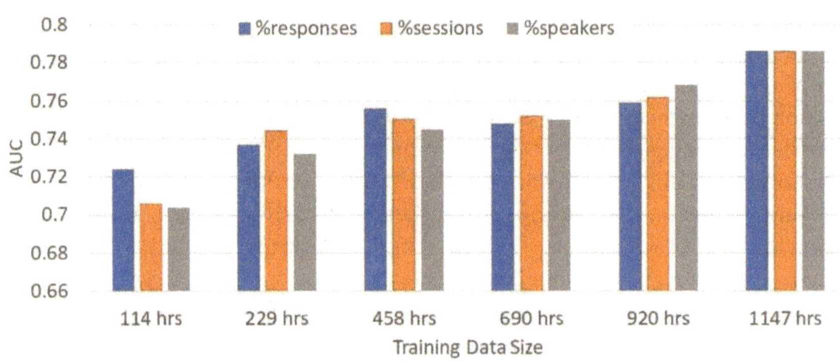

Fig. 5 AUC as a function of training data size. Size ranges from 10% (114 h) to 100% (1147 h)

length of 354 s). Figure 5 shows AUC performance as a function of the amount of training data. For each experiment, three trials (using three random subsets discussed above) are performed and then averaged to obtain the AUC value shown. Each experiment and trial uses data that was sampled independently, i.e. sampling with replacement.

From Fig. 5 and Table 6, several observations can be made. First, results improve almost linearly as more data is added, without performance saturation. Transfer learning provides significant gain across the range of corpus sizes, e.g., 15% gain for 10% of data. At the same time, adding more labeled data also improves model performance. For example, using all of the data (100%) results in 8% improvement relative to using 10% of the data.

Second, the 10%-responses subset has a higher AUC (0.725) relative to the 10%-sessions (0.706) and the 10%-speakers (0.704) subsets. This pattern of results suggests that, given a small amount of training data (here, less than 114 h), it is important to include a wide diversity of sessions and speakers. For example, almost 3% relative improvement in AUC can be obtained by trading session duration for a corresponding amount of speaking time from data representing a larger number of unique sessions and speakers. This gain can be observed in Fig. 5 as follows: in the first group of bars at 114 h of data, performance for the %sessions (orange) and %speakers (gray) is suppressed, compared with results for %responses (blue). The same pattern of suppressed performance is seen for regression results (not shown); in that case, for the 114-h subset, error metrics such as RMSE are raised for the %session and %speakers results.

Third, it is observed that using longer sessions during training provides only moderate performance gain. The AUC for the 10%-responses subset is 0.725. The average duration of sessions (output sessions after sampling) for this experiment is 45 s, and the number of independent sessions is 9032. The AUC for the 80%-sessions subset is 0.762, while the average duration of sessions is 354 s and the number of independent sessions is 9325. Ignoring the small difference between the number of independent sessions for these experiments (i.e., 9034 vs. 9325), the only major difference between these two experiments is the amount of speech data per session (i.e., session duration). By increasing the session duration from 45 s to 354 s (an 8$\times$ increase), only a 5% relative gain is obtained. These findings suggest that, for model training, relatively short sessions can be used without large degradation in performance. However, without adequate experimentation, this observation cannot be generalized to inference, nor to other models. For example, NLP models may be more sensitive than acoustic models to the length of training sessions.

4 NLP Models

4.1 Method

4.1.1 SVM Baseline Model

Learning word representations has been well known for many years. One of the most relevant approaches was based on building the representation in a vector space that enabled grouping of similar words together. Initial research for the SVM baseline model used word embeddings [77], an early method of NLP transfer learning. There are two main approaches: the Word2Vec method and the Glove method [78, 79]. Early analysis used Word2Vec, which can usually be trained using two methods as either a common bag of words or a skip-gram. The first is more suitable for large training sets.

In the latest transfer learning developments, the whole deep learning model, rather than particular layers, is used for further adaptation purposes. In the early days, the idea of Word2Vec was to use a particular layer of the network that would represent a given word. For a corpus of N words there would be the same number of vectors generated for further analysis.

Once the process of vectorizing words was complete, the SVM algorithm was used for classification training. There are various ways [80, 81] of combining vectors: average per session, p-mean, etc. For the SVM baseline model, the difference was not material whatsoever; all such approaches were roughly the same and inferior to the deep transfer learning methods described below.

4.1.2 Deep Learning Model

A recent focus in the NLP domain is to use the latest transfer learning methods [82] wherein the entire language model is used for classification purposes. Currently, the two most common topologies for language models encompass recurrent networks and transformers. Recurrent networks have been used very extensively in the models described in this chapter because, while they maintain very high accuracy, their topology has a smaller memory and computation footprint. Various methods can be used for tokenization purposes [83, 84]. In this deep learning model, the spaCy tokenization library is used; ultimately, each word is represented by a unique ID. The word dictionary used here contains over 20,000 individual tokens. Due to computing limitations and the time needed to train language models from scratch, the initial topology and tokenization technique were obtained from pretrained models. Figure 6 shows the entire flow of the NLP pipeline. As a next step, the training process included further pretraining of a generic language model on public data (see Sect. 2.1.3) that was specifically collected in order to emphasize emotion and mental health domain language structure. It was found that this approach stabilizes final depression predictions. At this stage, several language models were saved based on various hyper-parameters used to train them. Only at the end of the classification training process was the best language model identified. For example, language model performance metrics did not necessarily indicate the most optimal language model for the downstream task, e.g. some higher perplexity language models resulted in better classification results on our development test set.

The model used in this study is primarily based on LSTM topology inspired by the AWD-LSTM [85] architecture of the core language model and ULMFiT [86] work for model fine tuning. The approach is based on the following contributions. DropConnect, used for hidden-to-hidden layers, differs from the drop out approach by deactivating certain weights rather than activation mechanisms. Such an approach enables handling of the overfitting problem for RNNs while also allowing preservation of long-term dependencies. Another beneficial technique, back-propagation through time, dynamically changes the sequence length for the forward and backward passes. The third technique is embedding dropout, wherein occurrences of certain words are removed during the training stage. Averaged SGD is the last main component that improves model performance; it does so by

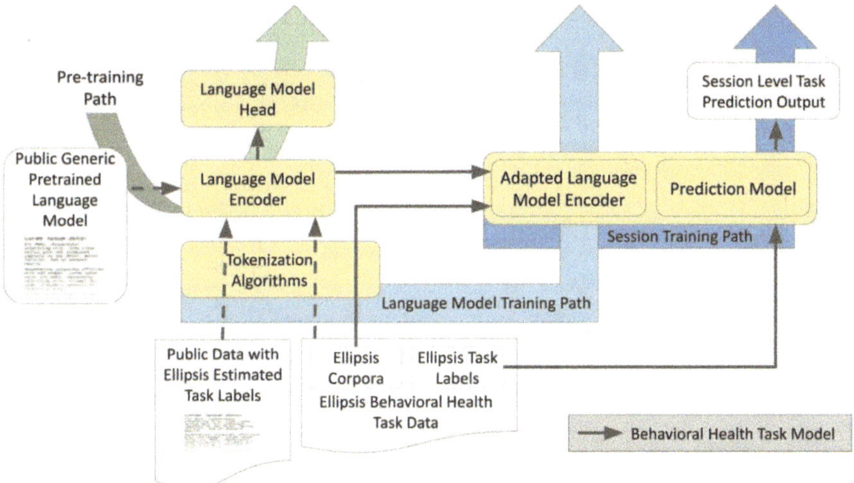

Fig. 6 An overview of the NLP model. Transfer learning is achieved using a language modeling task (dashed arrows)

averaging a number of previous iterations instead of taking SGD weight from the current iteration.

After the language model was trained on public corpora, an adaptation step based on proprietary data without labels was used to further train the Language Model encoder. As a next step, additional layers were added to the encoder for classification or regression purposes. The key mechanisms within this implementation encompass discriminative fine tuning, wherein the different layers of the network use different learning rates. This rate is the slanted triangular learning rate, in which the rate of change is dependent on the stage of the training process. The remaining main features cover gradual unfreezing and concatenated pooling of multiple time steps from the recurrent network.

4.2 *Experiments and Results*

4.2.1 Results for the General Population Corpus

This section presents the results of the NLP model for the General Population corpus. The model's behavior on subcategories of test sets is then described to demonstrate robustness under different conditions.

In this section, Deep Learning model performance for the General Population corpus described in Sect. 2.1.1 is reported. Given the use of large but proprietary datasets for both training and evaluation, it is useful to provide evidence of how the approaches described in this chapter perform on shared corpora. Due to lack of

Table 7 Regression results for depression prediction problem

Model	RMSE	MAE	PCC
NLP/GP dev	4.21	3.14	0.61
NLP/GP test	4.27	3.20	0.61
AVEC [47]/test	5.51	4.20	–

Table 8 Binary classification results for depression prediction

Model	AUC	Specificity at EER	Sensitivity at EER
NLP/GP dev	0.83	0.75	0.75
NLP/GP test	0.82	0.74	0.74
NLP/SP	0.76	0.69	0.69

access to benchmark corpora, indirect comparisons are provided. The comparisons are on different datasets, but, notably, both use PHQ-8 scores as the gold standard label. AVEC 2019 [14] was chosen as the comparison against which results are reported here for the NLP-based system only. Since Ringeval et al. [14] does not provide classification results, regression performance for the models is computed, and a RMSE metric used in Ringeval et al. [14] and elsewhere for the same data set is reported. RMSE is an error metric and is thus inversely correlated with performance. As shown in Table 7, the results for the NLP system demonstrate lower RMSE than the results for the system in Zhao et al. [47], again on different data. Table 8 provides standard binary classification results for both General Population and Senior Population test sets. It is believed that ROC AUC [87] is the best metric for this use case wherein the data is imbalanced and class separation is relevant. Table 8 also includes specificity and sensitivity at EER point.

Section 4.1.1 discussed SVM model performance as a simpler alternative to the deep learning models. The SVM model performance on the General Population corpus was AUC = 0.756, whereas performance for a single deep learning model was AUC = 0.828.

4.2.2 Results for the Senior Population Corpus

There is an important gap in the current literature with regard to how deep learning models generalize in the depression domain over different datasets. This chapter explores portability over two different corpora highly mismatched in age. Work presented in this chapter has been published in Rutowski et al. [88]. The first and larger corpus contained younger speakers and was used to train an NLP model to predict depression. As stated in Sect. 4.2.1, performance of AUC = 0.828 was obtained when testing on unseen speakers from the same age distribution. This model was then tested on the second corpus comprising seniors from a retirement community. Despite the large demographic differences in the two corpora, only modest degradation in performance for the senior data was observed, achieving AUC = 0.76. Interestingly, for the Senior Population corpus, performance for the

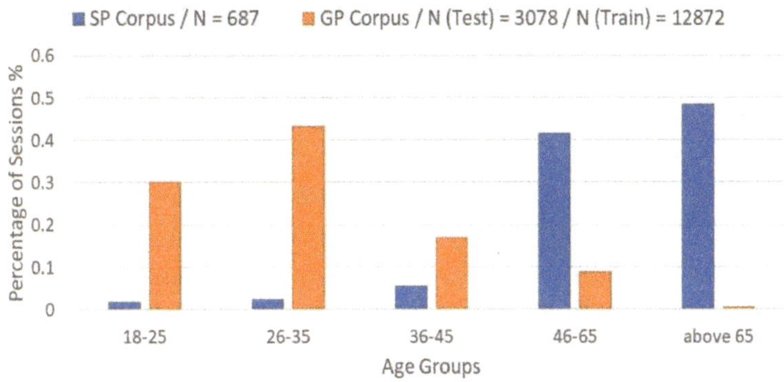

Fig. 7 Normalized age distribution for GP and SP corpus

subset of patients with consistent health state over time was AUC = 0.81. Implications for demographic portability of speech-based applications are discussed.

A striking difference in demographics between the corpora is age. As shown in Fig. 7, age distributions for the two corpora are largely non-overlapping. In this collection, most patients were expected to participate in a session once a week for 6 weeks. In the General Population collection, participation in more than one session was voluntary and could be conducted at any interval of at least 1 week. Repeated speakers in the General Population set were always placed only in the training partition. As shown in Table 1, the Senior Population dataset contains over 600 sessions. Senior Population sessions are shorter than the General Population sessions, containing on average 450 words vs. 800 words in General Population sessions. Thus, the mean number of responses is slightly higher (6.1 vs 5.2) for the Senior Population corpus. Given the size of the Senior Population corpus, it is used only for testing in this study. In addition to dep+ and dep− classes, a label dep+/− was introduced to subjects with two or more sessions who had at least one dep+ session and one dep− session. These patients are referred to as "inconsistent" (no judgment intended) with respect to depression class over time; patients with only same-class sessions over time are referred to as "consistent."

As described earlier, data labels represent PHQ-8 questionnaire results. Figure 2 shows the PHQ score label distribution of the General Population and Senior Population dataset. They are remarkably similar, with the lower rates at very low PHQ-8 scores being allocated somewhat evenly across the rest of the range. The prevalence differences are small (30% in Senior Population; 26.7% in General Population).

Figure 8 shows binary classification results for different test sets; the NLP system is always trained on the General Population corpus training data. GP indicates model performance when the General Population-trained model is tested on the separate General Population test set. SP indicates performance when the General Population model is tested on Senior Population data without retraining or tuning. As shown in the figure, there is a performance degradation (from .828 to .761) associated with

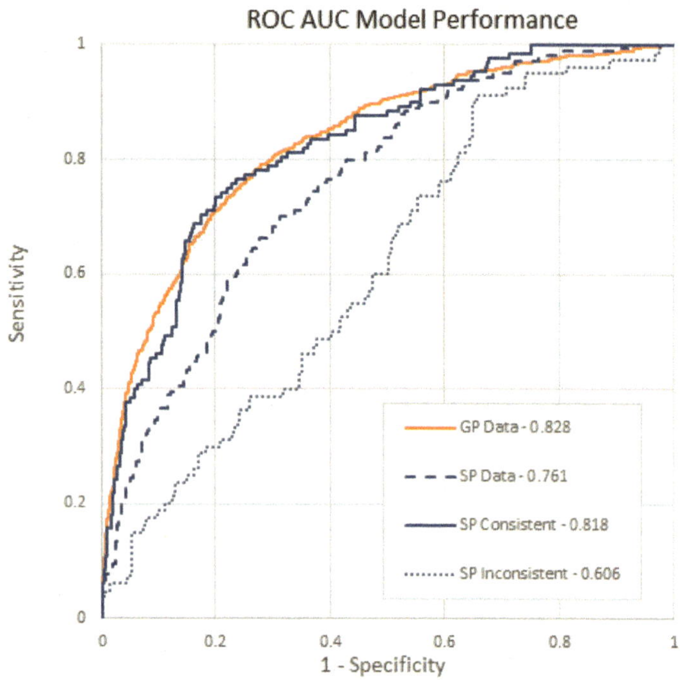

Fig. 8 AUC performance on various test sets for NLP model. The model is always trained on the GP training set

the mismatch. Given the major age distribution difference, this is a better result than expected. It suggests that patterns captured by the language model as indicators of depression may be largely portable across these age groups without need for significant retraining.

In the Senior Population test corpus, patients participated in a longitudinal study as described earlier. Interestingly, classification performance of the General Population-trained NLP model depends strongly on consistency of a patient's self-reported PHQ-8 scores over the multiple-session collection (with sessions roughly 1 week apart on average). Out of 161 unique patients in the Senior Population corpus, 124 had PHQ-8 scores that were either always dep+ or always dep− over their sessions. The remaining 37 patients had a mix (dep+/−) of sessions over the course of their collection. The mean number of responses per session over the full SP set was 6.1, as shown in Table 1; for the longitudinal patients, the mean number of responses per session was 4.2. Interestingly, a large difference in the number of responses per session was found between consistent and inconsistent longitudinal SP users. The difference is not correlated with depression class. Consistent users averaged 3.8 responses, whereas inconsistent users averaged 5.5. This difference is relevant to the design of future speech elicitation applications.

Overall, consistent patients were more concise and had fewer responses than inconsistent patients. Figure 8 reveals a marked difference in model performance as a function of user consistency even though each session is treated independently. Performance for consistent SP patients is 0.82 versus 0.61 for inconsistent SP patients. Despite the large mismatch in age as well as other factors in the two corpora, the model surprisingly performed about as well on mismatched-age (SP) consistent users as on matched-age (GP) users. It is intended that future work will investigate the role of longitudinal consistency. What is clear is that there is good portability in the NLP model, especially for consistent patients.

5 General Analysis

In Fig. 9, the AUC curve of the NLP and acoustic models are compared using the performance of primary care providers (PCPs) as reference points. Here, the results of a single LSTM NLP model and a single acoustic + TL model are shown. Data points from three separate studies of PCPs are included as reference points. These data reflect results on depression detection performance by PCPs not specifically trained in mental health assessment. Note that these studies are not directly comparable to ours nor to each other due to differences in data and methods used. They do, however, provide a crude indication of human performance in the context of a general PCP visit [6, 89, 90].

Table 9 shows the results for the acoustic and NLP models on subsets of the test data broken down by metadata categories: session count of train and test sets, depression rate in test set sessions, and mean PHQ-8 score of test set sessions. These results are also published in our previous paper [48]. Notice that since each session in the test set is contributed by a unique user previously unseen in the train set, the depression rate of the test session and the mean PHQ-8 of test sessions is the same as the depression rate of the test population and mean PHQ-8 of the test population. To avoid noisy results, categories with session counts below 150 are excluded.

The following observations can be made from Table 9. Overall, both acoustic and NLP models are robust over speaker characteristics. There are some exceptions, as indicated by entries marked with an asterisk. A marked entry indicates that the AUC of the category is significantly higher or lower than that of other members in the metadata group with $p < 0.05$.

For the acoustic model, performance on depression classification is significantly lower if the speaker is age 26–35 or identifies as Hispanic. There are no such differences for the NLP model. Metadata on user location was also collected because it is correlated with other factors such as socioeconomic status, regional accents (relevant to ASR), and other variables. The rate of depression is similar across locations but there are performance differences. It is premature to propose reasons for this, but this set is included to demonstrate that not all variables result in similar performance.

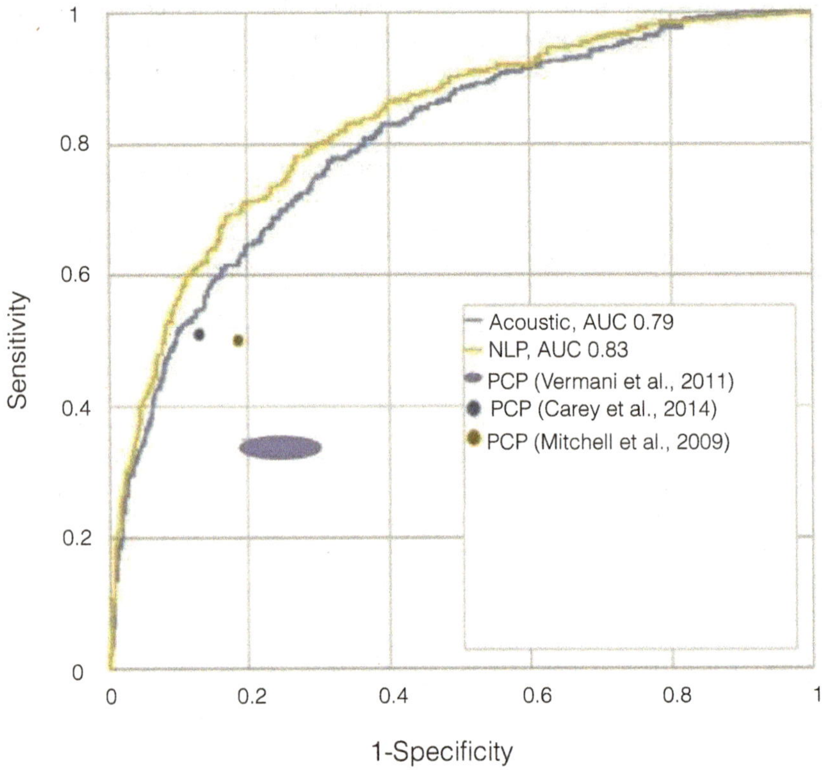

Fig. 9 ROC curves for single acoustic and NLP models. For reference, results from human PCP studies [6, 89, 90] are shown but are not directly comparable due to differences in data and models used

Overall, both models are remarkably consistent. They discriminate between positive and negative depression classes at a level that is not significantly different from the other members of the set and is similar to the overall performance level of the full test set, as shown in Table 9. Despite differences in priors and in PHQ-8 distributions, the ability of the models to separate classes does not change significantly for most user conditions, including gender, smoking, and marital status. The AUC of the 26–35 age group is slightly lower than that of the rest of the population and this difference is statistically significant. This result is currently being investigated; given that this group has a large amount of training data, data sparsity is not a concern.

Additionally, both models' AUCs are robust over session metadata regarding temporal information of user recording time, including local time of day, day of week, and season. For example, in Fig. 3, changes in PHQ-8 average can be seen over the course of the day, but the AUC for depression detection does not change significantly over this factor. Both models are largely robust to other time-

Table 9 Model performance by test subset

	Metadata	Categories	Train set sessions count	Test set sessions count	Depression rate	Mean PHQ [a]	Acoustic AUC	NLP AUC
Base performance over all test sets			11,620	3078	25.7%	5.93	0.779	0.825
User metadata	Gender	Male	3125	1244	20.4%	5.74	0.769	0.819
		Female	4419	1790	35.3%	6.77	0.774	0.820
	Age group	18–25	2087	847	30.0%	7.32	0.792	0.828
		26–35	3256	1382	24.8%	6.40	0.752*	0.820
		36–45	1444	513	18.7%	5.60	0.790	0.808
		46–65	766	283	34.6%	4.78	0.792	0.819
	Smoking	Non-smoker	3850	813	23.2%	6.44	0.803	0.836
		Smoker	1807	397	31.3%	7.47	0.767	0.808
	U.S. States (selected)	California	924	266	26.8%	6.68	0.741	0.830
		Florida	831	253	26.2%	6.41	0.842*	0.875*
		Texas	723	232	26.0%	6.66	0.810	0.845
		New York	596	142	25.7%	6.70	0.815	0.887*
	Ethnicity	Caucasian	5219	2039	24.7%	6.05	0.796	0.826
		African American	569	241	19.7%	5.63	0.777	0.812
		Hispanic	552	248	25.0%	6.73	0.676*	0.788
		Asian American	452	185	20.0%	5.61	0.789	0.841
		Mixed	364	173	31.3%	7.22	0.768	0.827

(continued)

Table 9 (continued)

	Metadata	Categories	Train set sessions count	Test set sessions count	Depression rate	Mean PHQ [a]	Acoustic AUC	NLP AUC
	Marital	Never married	1850	188	31.5%	7.84	0.778	0.857
		Married	1220	173	21.2%	5.20	0.774	0.829
Session Metadata	Time of day[b]	Morning	1275	476	24.3%	6.39	0.785	0.823
		Afternoon	3471	1127	22.7%	6.08	0.776	0.841
		Night	4012	1005	26.3%	6.76	0.783	0.815
		Late night	2457	472	31.2%	7.26	0.758	0.804
	Day of week	Weekdays	9343	2307	25.2%	6.54	0.782	0.832
		Weekends	1872	773	27.5%	6.88	0.772	0.802
	Time of year[c]	Summer	993	756	20.1%	5.39	0.818	0.838
		Rest of the year	6056	2324	27.0%	6.88	0.769	0.821

* $p < 0.05$ in statistical significance test of AUC [59]. The denoted category has a significantly different AUC than others in same set

[a] The mean PHQ is calculated using only the first session for each speaker in the designated subset to avoid skewing of mean PHQ by speakers who participated multiple times. For most speakers, the first session was their only session

[b] We partitioned the day into four 6-h parts for analysis: morning is defined as 6 am to noon, afternoon as noon to 6 pm, night as 6 pm to midnight, and late night as midnight to 6 am. Time is local for the user. Other session factors such as day of week and month of year also showed effects but are not shown due to space restrictions

[c] Summer is defined as the time of year where the month is June, July, or August

related session variables, including time of day, day of week, and time of year. This performance consistency holds despite differences across categories in PHQ-8 priors.

6 Summary, Conclusions and Future Work

In this chapter, acoustic and NLP models for predicting depression from speech were investigated using a large depression-labeled corpus. Results showed excellent performance overall with respect to generalization over different demographic groups, which is important when a screening tool is deployed to screen a diverse population.

Acoustic models and applications of transfer learning to improve the performance of models are explored thoroughly in this chapter. A transfer learning scheme proposed in this chapter based on an ASR source task resulted in a 27% relative performance boost for binary classification and a 10–15% relative reduction in regression error metrics relative to baseline models without transfer learning. Experiments also show that transfer learning works even when the performance of the source task (e.g. ASR) is poor. It is hypothesized that the restrictions imposed by source tasks on learnable parameters are the main reason that transfer learning performs so well in this problem, as opposed to e.g., learning how to transcribe speech. This hypothesis requires further investigation for which future experiments are planned. Furthermore, it is intended that future work will study the effect of source task performance, source task type (e.g., unsupervised tasks), and source task data.

The effect of the training dataset size on classification performance was also investigated by subsampling from the large training corpus. Subsamples were created using different data units, including responses, sessions, and speakers. Overall, it was found that adding training data results in roughly linear gains in performance, and that even at 1200 h of training data, the acoustic + TL model does not show signs of saturation. It was found that, even for the smallest data subset (114 h or 10% of the training set), the addition of transfer learning led to a sizeable (15%) gain in AUC relative to a model trained with 100% of the labeled data but no transfer learning. In addition, it was found that for smaller training data subsets (under about 100 h), diversity of sessions and speakers is important. In such cases, session duration is not as important as the number of independent sessions or speakers. More work is needed to assess a minimum viable session duration for this finding because extremely short sessions may not provide any value in training.

In addition, a state-of-the-art depression classifier based on deep NLP and transfer learning showed excellent portability over age, gender, and ethnicity. Using two corpora almost non-overlapping in age but similar in collection design, only a small degradation in binary classification performance (0.06 absolute AUC) was found when testing speakers mismatched for age. Interestingly, this degradation nearly disappeared for those seniors reporting consistent class labels over their longitudinal samples. Furthermore, many other experiments were performed which have been omitted from this chapter. One such relevant study investigated the effect of speech length during inference time [15], finding that the performance of the NLP model degrades once session length is less than 2 min. Therefore, for any clinical deployment, it is suggested that session length should be at least approximately 2 min or 120 words [15].

Robust results were obtained with no difference in performance between test and development sets. Models introduced in this chapter were trained on a large dataset of about 10,000 unique speakers and 1600 h of speech. This allowed for the investigation of the robustness of these models relative to different independent factors, including user demographics and recording environments. Model performance was measured on different subsets of test data without model retraining or optimization for each subset. Results showed that both acoustic and NLP models generalize well over different factors, with some small exceptions for acoustic models. This pattern holds despite the differences in priors for both category frequencies and PHQ-8 value distributions of metadata categories. The robustness of both models further demonstrates that those deep learning models trained on a fixed set of samples will generalize over specific speaker and temporal variables in unseen data, both from comparable and from completely different demographics. Future works should examine additional types of metadata such as recording quality, ASR quality, recording device usage, etc.

A natural next step is to explore the fusion of these models to generate predictions based on both acoustic and text modalities. It is expected that proper fusion algorithms will improve the performance and robustness of these models. Another important direction of investigation is the interpretability of predictions. Deep learning models such as the ones explored in this chapter work as black boxes and, little insight can be gained by only observing the predictions made. In order to make these predictions more useful for clinical applications, some type of interpretability and explainability is desired.

Finally, as mentioned in the introduction, the robustness analysis in this chapter is a start but is limited because only subsets within a matched collection are examined. It is critical to examine corpora with large demographic differences as well as with differences in how speech is collected by an application, ideally with clinical labels (as opposed to self-administered tests such as PHQ). This is the ultimate goal of Ellipsis Health and is currently under investigation.

Acknowledgments This paper and the research behind it would not have been possible without the exceptional support of the Ellipsis Health team. We specially thank our clinical team: Mike Aratow, Farshid Haque, Tahmida Nazreen and Melissa McCool. We thank Mainul Mondal and Susan Solinsky for their continuing support. Additionally, we thank Vanessa Lin and Nina Roth for editing the manuscript for this chapter.

References

1. Otte, C., Gold, S. M., Penninx, B. W., Pariante, C. M., Etkin, A., Fava, M., Mohr, D. C., & Schatzberg, A. F. (2016). Major depressive disorder. *Nature Reviews Disease Primers, 2*(1), 16065. https://doi.org/10.1038/nrdp.2016.65
2. World Health Organisation. (2017). *Depression and other common mental disorders: Global health estimates*. World Health Organization.
3. NIH. (2019, February). *Major depression*. Retrieved January 22, 2021, from https://www.nimh.nih.gov/health/statistics/major-depression.shtml.
4. *Depression*. (n.d.). Centers for Disease Control and Prevention. Retrieved January 22, 2021, from https://www.cdc.gov/nchs/fastats/depression.htm.
5. Kuhl, E. A. (2018). *Quantifying the cost of depression*. Center For Workplace Mental Health. Retrieved from http://www.workplacementalhealth.org/Mental-Health-Topics/Depression/Quantifying-the-Cost-of-Depression.
6. Mitchell, A. J., Vaze, A., & Rao, S. (2009). Clinical diagnosis of depression in primary care: A meta-analysis. *The Lancet, 374*(9690), 609–619. https://doi.org/10.1016/S0140-6736(09)60879-5
7. Simon, G. E., VonKorff, M., Piccinelli, M., Fullerton, C., & Ormel, J. (1999). An international study of the relation between somatic symptoms and depression. *New England Journal of Medicine, 341*(18), 1329–1335. https://doi.org/10.1056/NEJM199910283411801
8. Nease, D. E., & Maloin, J. M. (2003). Depression screening: A practical strategy. *The Journal of Family Practice, 52*(2), 118–124. http://www.ncbi.nlm.nih.gov/pubmed/12585989.
9. Resnik, P., Garron, A., & Resnik, R. (2013). Using topic modeling to improve prediction of neuroticism and depression in college students. In *EMNLP 2013—2013 conference on empirical methods in natural language processing, proceedings of the conference*, pp. 1348–1353.
10. Cummins, N., Scherer, S., Krajewski, J., Schnieder, S., Epps, J., & Quatieri, T. F. (2015). A review of depression and suicide risk assessment using speech analysis. *Speech Communication, 71*, 10–49. https://doi.org/10.1016/j.specom.2015.03.004
11. Williamson, J. R., Godoy, E., Cha, M., Schwarzentruber, A., Khorrami, P., Gwon, Y., Kung, H.-T., Dagli, C., & Quatieri, T. F. (2016). Detecting depression using vocal, facial and semantic communication cues. In *Proceedings of the 6th international workshop on audio/visual emotion challenge*, pp. 11–18. https://doi.org/10.1145/2988257.2988263.
12. Pampouchidou, A., Simantiraki, O., Fazlollahi, A., Pediaditis, M., Manousos, D., Roniotis, A., Giannakakis, G., Meriaudeau, F., Simos, P., Marias, K., Yang, F., & Tsiknakis, M. (2016). Depression assessment by fusing high and low level features from audio, video, and text. *Proceedings of the 6th international workshop on audio/visual emotion challenge*, pp. 27–34. https://doi.org/10.1145/2988257.2988266.
13. Yang, L., Sahli, H., Xia, X., Pei, E., Oveneke, M. C., & Jiang, D. (2017). Hybrid depression classification and estimation from audio video and text information. In *Proceedings of the 7th annual workshop on audio/visual emotion challenge*, pp. 45–51. https://doi.org/10.1145/3133944.3133950.
14. Ringeval, F., Messner, E.-M., Song, S., Liu, S., Zhao, Z., Mallol-Ragolta, A., Ren, Z., Soleymani, M., Pantic, M., Schuller, B., Valstar, M., Cummins, N., Cowie, R., Tavabi, L., Schmitt, M., Alisamir, S., & Amiriparian, S. (2019). AVEC 2019 workshop and challenge: State-of-mind, detecting depression with AI, and cross-cultural affect recognition. In *Proceedings of the 9th international on audio/visual emotion challenge and workshop—AVEC '19*, pp. 3–12. https://doi.org/10.1145/3347320.3357688.

15. Rutowski, T., Harati, A., Lu, Y., & Shriberg, E. (2019). Optimizing speech-input length for speaker-independent depression classification. *Interspeech, 2019*, 3023–3027. https://doi.org/10.21437/Interspeech.2019-3095
16. Cohn, J. F., Cummins, N., Epps, J., Goecke, R., Joshi, J., & Scherer, S. (2018). Multimodal assessment of depression from behavioral signals. In *The handbook of multimodal-multisensor interfaces: Foundations, user modeling, and common modality combinations—Volume 2* (pp. 375–417). Association for Computing Machinery. https://doi.org/10.1145/3107990.3108004
17. Scherer, S., Stratou, G., Gratch, J., & Morency, L. P. (2013). Investigating voice quality as a speaker-independent indicator of depression and PTSD. In *Proceedings of the annual conference of the International Speech Communication Association, INTERSPEECH*, pp. 847–851.
18. Helfer, B. S., Quatieri, T. F., Williamson, J. R., Mehta, D. D., Horwitz, R., & Yu, B. (2013). Classification of depression state based on articulatory precision. In *Proceedings of the annual conference of the International Speech Communication Association, INTERSPEECH*, pp. 2172–2176.
19. Stasak, B., Epps, J., & Goecke, R. (2019). An investigation of linguistic stress and articulatory vowel characteristics for automatic depression classification. *Computer Speech & Language, 53*, 140–155. https://doi.org/10.1016/j.csl.2018.08.001
20. Trevino, A. C., Quatieri, T. F., & Malyska, N. (2011). Phonologically-based biomarkers for major depressive disorder. *EURASIP Journal on Advances in Signal Processing, 2011*(1), 42. https://doi.org/10.1186/1687-6180-2011-42
21. Horwitz, R., Quatieri, T. F., Helfer, B. S., Yu, B., Williamson, J. R., & Mundt, J. (2013). On the relative importance of vocal source, system, and prosody in human depression. In *2013 IEEE international conference on body sensor networks*, pp. 1–6. https://doi.org/10.1109/BSN.2013.6575522.
22. Sacks, H. (1995). *Lectures on conversation*. Wiley-Blackwell. https://doi.org/10.1002/9781444328301
23. Pennebaker, J. W., Mehl, M. R., & Niederhoffer, K. G. (2003). Psychological aspects of natural language use: Our words, our selves. *Annual Review of Psychology, 54*(1), 547–577. https://doi.org/10.1146/annurev.psych.54.101601.145041
24. Pestian, J. P., Matykiewicz, P., Linn-Gust, M., South, B., Uzuner, O., Wiebe, J., Cohen, K. B., Hurdle, J., & Brew, C. (2012). Sentiment analysis of suicide notes: A shared task. *Biomedical Informatics Insights, 5*, BII-S9042. https://doi.org/10.4137/BII.S9042
25. Ramirez-Esparza, N., Chung, C. K., Kacewicz, E., & Pennebaker, J. W. (2008). *The psychology of word use in depression forums in English and in Spanish: Testing two text analytic approaches*. Retrieved from www.aaai.org.
26. Huang, S. H., LePendu, P., Iyer, S. V., Tai-Seale, M., Carrell, D., & Shah, N. H. (2014a). Toward personalizing treatment for depression: Predicting diagnosis and severity. *Journal of the American Medical Informatics Association, 21*(6), 1069–1075. https://doi.org/10.1136/amiajnl-2014-002733
27. Perlis, R. H., Iosifescu, D. V., Castro, V. M., Murphy, S. N., Gainer, V. S., Minnier, J., Cai, T., Goryachev, S., Zeng, Q., Gallagher, P. J., Fava, M., Weilburg, J. B., Churchill, S. E., Kohane, I. S., & Smoller, J. W. (2012). Using electronic medical records to enable large-scale studies in psychiatry: Treatment resistant depression as a model. *Psychological Medicine, 42*(1), 41–50. https://doi.org/10.1017/S0033291711000997
28. Cook, B. L., Progovac, A. M., Chen, P., Mullin, B., Hou, S., & Baca-Garcia, E. (2016). Novel use of Natural Language Processing (NLP) to predict suicidal ideation and psychiatric symptoms in a text-based mental health intervention in Madrid. *Computational and Mathematical Methods in Medicine, 2016*, 8708434. https://doi.org/10.1155/2016/8708434
29. Yates, A., Cohan, A., & Goharian, N. (2017). Depression and self-harm risk assessment in online forums. In *Proceedings of the 2017 conference on empirical methods in natural language processing*, pp. 2968–2978. https://doi.org/10.18653/v1/D17-1322.

30. Chan, W., Jaitly, N., Le, Q., & Vinyals, O. (2016). Listen, attend and spell: A neural network for large vocabulary conversational speech recognition. *2016 IEEE international conference on acoustics, speech and signal processing (ICASSP)*, pp. 4960–4964. https://doi.org/10.1109/ICASSP.2016.7472621.
31. Kim, S., Hori, T., & Watanabe, S. (2017). Joint CTC-attention based end-to-end speech recognition using multi-task learning. In *2017 IEEE international conference on acoustics, speech and signal processing (ICASSP)*, pp. 4835–4839. https://doi.org/10.1109/ICASSP.2017.7953075.
32. Narayanan, A., Prabhavalkar, R., Chiu, C.-C., Rybach, D., Sainath, T. N., & Strohman, T. (2019). Recognizing long-form speech using streaming end-to-end models. In *2019 IEEE automatic speech recognition and understanding workshop (ASRU)*, pp. 920–927. https://doi.org/10.1109/ASRU46091.2019.9003913.
33. Deng, J., Zhang, Z., Marchi, E., & Schuller, B. (2013). Sparse autoencoder-based feature transfer learning for speech emotion recognition. In *2013 Humaine association conference on affective computing and intelligent interaction*, pp. 511–516. https://doi.org/10.1109/ACII.2013.90.
34. Huang, Z., Dong, M., Mao, Q., & Zhan, Y. (2014b). Speech emotion recognition using CNN. In *Proceedings of the 22nd ACM international conference on multimedia*, pp. 801–804. https://doi.org/10.1145/2647868.2654984.
35. Huang, Z., Epps, J., & Joachim, D. (2020). Exploiting vocal tract coordination using dilated CNNS for depression detection in naturalistic environments. In *ICASSP 2020—2020 IEEE international conference on acoustics, speech and signal processing (ICASSP)*, pp. 6549–6553. https://doi.org/10.1109/ICASSP40776.2020.9054323.
36. Kahou, S. E., Bouthillier, X., Lamblin, P., Gulcehre, C., Michalski, V., Konda, K., Jean, S., Froumenty, P., Dauphin, Y., Boulanger-Lewandowski, N., Chandias Ferrari, R., Mirza, M., Warde-Farley, D., Courville, A., Vincent, P., Memisevic, R., Pal, C., & Bengio, Y. (2016). EmoNets: Multimodal deep learning approaches for emotion recognition in video. *Journal on Multimodal User Interfaces, 10*(2), 99–111. https://doi.org/10.1007/s12193-015-0195-2
37. Lim, W., Jang, D., & Lee, T. (2016). Speech emotion recognition using convolutional and recurrent neural networks. In *2016 Asia-Pacific Signal and Information Processing Association annual summit and conference (APSIPA)*, pp. 1–4. doi:https://doi.org/10.1109/APSIPA.2016.7820699.
38. Mao, Q., Dong, M., Huang, Z., & Zhan, Y. (2014). Learning salient features for speech emotion recognition using convolutional neural networks. *IEEE Transactions on Multimedia, 16*(8), 2203–2213. https://doi.org/10.1109/TMM.2014.2360798
39. Yang, L., Jiang, D., & Sahli, H. (2020). Feature augmenting networks for improving depression severity estimation from speech signals. *IEEE Access, 8*, 24033–24045. https://doi.org/10.1109/ACCESS.2020.2970496
40. He, L., & Cao, C. (2018). Automated depression analysis using convolutional neural networks from speech. *Journal of Biomedical Informatics, 83*, 103–111. https://doi.org/10.1016/j.jbi.2018.05.007
41. Coutinho, E., Deng, J., & Schuller, B. (2014). Transfer learning emotion manifestation across music and speech. *International Joint Conference on Neural Networks (IJCNN), 2014*, 3592–3598. https://doi.org/10.1109/IJCNN.2014.6889814
42. Coutinho, E., & Schuller, B. (2017). Shared acoustic codes underlie emotional communication in music and speech—Evidence from deep transfer learning. *PLoS One, 12*(6), e0179289. https://doi.org/10.1371/journal.pone.0179289
43. Li, Q., & Chaspari, T. (2019). Exploring transfer learning between scripted and spontaneous speech for emotion recognition. In *2019 international conference on multimodal interaction*, pp. 435–439. https://doi.org/10.1145/3340555.3353762.
44. Du, W., Morency, L.-P., Cohn, J., & Black, A. W. (2019). Bag-of-acoustic-words for mental health assessment: A deep autoencoding approach. *Interspeech, 2019*, 1428–1432. https://doi.org/10.21437/Interspeech.2019-3059

45. Martinez-Castaño, R., Htait, A., Azzopardi, L., & Moshfeghi, Y. (2020). Early risk detection of self-harm and depression severity using BERT-based transformers: iLab at CLEF eRisk 2020. *CEUR Workshop Proceedings*, 2696.
46. Salekin, A., Eberle, J. W., Glenn, J. J., Teachman, B. A., & Stankovic, J. A. (2018). A weakly supervised learning framework for detecting social anxiety and depression. *Proceedings of the ACM on Interactive, Mobile, Wearable and Ubiquitous Technologies, 2*(2), 1–26. https://doi.org/10.1145/3214284
47. Zhao, Z., Bao, Z., Zhang, Z., Deng, J., Cummins, N., Wang, H., Tao, J., & Schuller, B. (2020). Automatic assessment of depression from speech via a hierarchical attention transfer network and attention autoencoders. *IEEE Journal of Selected Topics in Signal Processing, 14*(2), 423–434. https://doi.org/10.1109/JSTSP.2019.2955012
48. Lu, Y., Harati, A., Rutowski, T., Oliveira, R., Chlebek, P., & Shriberg, E. (2020). Robust speech and natural language processing models for depression screening. In *The 2020 IEEE signal processing in medicine and biology symposium*, pp. 1–5.
49. Valstar, M., Gratch, J., Schuller, B., Ringeval, F., Lalanne, D., Torres Torres, M., Scherer, S., Stratou, G., Cowie, R., & Pantic, M. (2016). AVEC 2016: Depression, mood, and emotion recognition workshop and challenge. In *Proceedings of the 6th international workshop on audio/visual emotion challenge*, pp. 3–10. https://doi.org/10.1145/2988257.2988258.
50. Valstar, M., Schuller, B., Smith, K., Almaev, T., Eyben, F., Krajewski, J., Cowie, R., & Pantic, M. (2014). AVEC 2014: 3D dimensional affect and depression recognition challenge. In *Proceedings of the 4th international workshop on audio/visual emotion challenge—AVEC '14*, pp. 3–10. https://doi.org/10.1145/2661806.2661807.
51. Stasak, B., Epps, J., & Goecke, R. (2017). Elicitation design for acoustic depression classification: An investigation of articulation effort, linguistic complexity, and word affect. In *Proceedings of the annual conference of the international speech communication association, INTERSPEECH*, pp. 834–838. https://doi.org/10.21437/Interspeech.2017-1223.
52. Jiahong, Y., Liberman, M., & Cieri, C. (2006). Towards an integrated understanding of speaking rate in conversation. *Proceedings of the Annual Conference of the International Speech Communication Association, INTERSPEECH, 2*, 541–544.
53. Kroenke, K., Strine, T. W., Spitzer, R. L., Williams, J. B. W., Berry, J. T., & Mokdad, A. H. (2009). The PHQ-8 as a measure of current depression in the general population. *Journal of Affective Disorders, 114*(1–3), 163–173. https://doi.org/10.1016/j.jad.2008.06.026
54. National population by characteristics: 2010–2019. (n.d.). Retrieved from https://www.census.gov/data/tables/time-series/demo/popest/2010s-national-detail.html.
55. ACS demographic and housing estimates—2011–2015. (n.d.). Retrieved from https://www.census.gov/programs-surveys/acs/technical-documentation/table-and-geography-changes/2015/5-year.html.
56. Merity, S., Xiong, C., Bradbury, J., & Socher, R. (2016). Pointer sentinel mixture models. In *5th international conference on learning representations, ICLR 2017—Conference track proceedings*. http://arxiv.org/abs/1609.07843.
57. Schwenk, H., Wenzek, G., Edunov, S., Grave, E., & Joulin, A. (2019). *CCMatrix: Mining billions of high-quality parallel sentences on the WEB*. CoRR, abs/1911.0. Retrieved from http://arxiv.org/abs/1911.04944.
58. Panayotov, V., Chen, G., Povey, D., & Khudanpur, S. (2015). Librispeech: An ASR corpus based on public domain audio books. In *2015 IEEE international conference on acoustics, speech and signal processing (ICASSP)*, pp. 5206–5210. https://doi.org/10.1109/ICASSP.2015.7178964.
59. DeLong, E. R., DeLong, D. M., & Clarke-Pearson, D. L. (1988). Comparing the areas under two or more correlated receiver operating characteristic curves: A nonparametric approach. *Biometrics, 44*(3), 837. https://doi.org/10.2307/2531595
60. Sun, X., & Xu, W. (2014). Fast implementation of DeLong's algorithm for comparing the areas under correlated receiver operating characteristic curves. *IEEE Signal Processing Letters, 21*(11), 1389–1393. https://doi.org/10.1109/LSP.2014.2337313

61. Mundt, J. C., Snyder, P. J., Cannizzaro, M. S., Chappie, K., & Geralts, D. S. (2007). Voice acoustic measures of depression severity and treatment response collected via interactive voice response (IVR) technology. *Journal of Neurolinguistics, 20*(1), 50–64. https://doi.org/10.1016/j.jneuroling.2006.04.001
62. Ray, A., Kumar, S., Reddy, R., Mukherjee, P., & Garg, R. (2019). Multi-level attention network using text, audio and video for depression prediction. In *Proceedings of the 9th international on audio/visual emotion challenge and workshop—AVEC '19*, pp. 81–88. https://doi.org/10.1145/3347320.3357697.
63. Paszke, A., Gross, S., Massa, F., Lerer, A., Bradbury, J., Chanan, G., Killeen, T., Lin, Z., Gimelshein, N., Antiga, L., Desmaison, A., Köpf, A., Yang, E., DeVito, Z., Raison, M., Tejani, A., Chilamkurthy, S., Steiner, B., Fang, L., ... Chintala, S. (2019). PyTorch: An imperative style, high-performance deep learning library. *Advances in Neural Information Processing Systems.*
64. Glorot, X., Bordes, A., & Bengio, Y. (2011). Domain adaptation for large-scale sentiment classification: A deep learning approach. In *Proceedings of the 28th international conference on machine learning, ICML 2011*, pp. 513–520.
65. Caruana, R. (1997). Multitask learning. *Machine Learning, 28*(1), 41–75. https://doi.org/10.1023/A:1007379606734
66. Zadeh, L. M., Silbert, N. H., Sternasty, K., Swanepoel, D. W., Hunter, L. L., & Moore, D. R. (2019). Extended high-frequency hearing enhances speech perception in noise. *Proceedings of the National Academy of Sciences of the United States of America.*https://doi.org/10.1073/pnas.1903315116
67. Lüke, H. D. (1999). The origins of the sampling theorem. *IEEE Communications Magazine, 37*(4), 106–108. https://doi.org/10.1109/35.755459
68. Ravindran, S., Demiroglu, C., & Anderson, D. V. (2003). Speech recognition using filter-bank features. In *The thirty-seventh Asilomar conference on signals, systems & computers, 2003*, pp. 1900–1903. https://doi.org/10.1109/ACSSC.2003.1292312.
69. Ravi, V., Fan, R., Afshan, A., Lu, H., & Alwan, A. (2020). Exploring the use of an unsupervised autoregressive model as a shared encoder for text-dependent speaker verification. *Interspeech, 2020*, 766–770. https://doi.org/10.21437/Interspeech.2020-2957
70. Parthasarathy, S., & Busso, C. (2018). Ladder networks for emotion recognition: Using unsupervised auxiliary tasks to improve predictions of emotional attributes. *Interspeech, 2018*, 3698–3702. https://doi.org/10.21437/Interspeech.2018-1391
71. Liu, A. H., Sung, T.-W., Chuang, S.-P., Lee, H., & Lee, L. (2020). Sequence-to-sequence automatic speech recognition with word embedding regularization and fused decoding. In *ICASSP 2020—2020 IEEE international conference on acoustics, speech and signal processing (ICASSP)*, pp. 7879–7883. https://doi.org/10.1109/ICASSP40776.2020.9053324.
72. Simonyan, K., & Zisserman, A. (2015). Very deep convolutional networks for large-scale image recognition. In *3rd international conference on learning representations, ICLR 2015—Conference track proceedings.*
73. Graves, A., & Schmidhuber, J. (2005). Framewise phoneme classification with bidirectional LSTM and other neural network architectures. *Neural Networks, 18*(5–6), 602–610. https://doi.org/10.1016/j.neunet.2005.06.042
74. Lai, S., Xu, L., Liu, K., & Zhao, J. (2015). Recurrent convolutional neural networks for text classification. In *Proceedings of the national conference on artificial intelligence*, pp. 2267–2273.
75. Harati, A., Shriberg, E., Rutowski, T., Chlebek, P., Lu, Y., & Oliveira, R. (2021). Speech-based depression prediction using encoder-weight-only transfer learning and a large corpus. In *ICASSP 2021—2021 IEEE international conference on acoustics, speech and signal processing (ICASSP)*, pp. 7273–7277.
76. Al Hanai, T., Ghassemi, M., & Glass, J. (2018). Detecting depression with audio/text sequence modeling of interviews. *Interspeech, 2018*, 1716–1720. https://doi.org/10.21437/Interspeech.2018-2522

77. Bengio, Y., Ducharme, R., & Vincent, P. (2001). A neural probabilistic language model. *Advances in Neural Information Processing Systems, 3*, 1137–1155.
78. Mikolov, T., Sutskever, I., Chen, K., Corrado, G. S., & Dean, J. (2013). Distributed representations of words and phrases and their compositionality. In C. J. C. Burges, L. Bottou, M. Welling, Z. Ghahramani, & K. Q. Weinberger (Eds.), *Advances in neural information processing systems* (Vol. 26, pp. 3111–3119). Curran Associates. https://proceedings.neurips.cc/paper/2013/file/9aa42b31882ec039965f3c4923ce901b-Paper.pdf.
79. Pennington, J., Socher, R., & Manning, C. D. (2014). GloVe: Global vectors for word representation. In *EMNLP 2014—2014 conference on empirical methods in natural language processing, proceedings of the conference*, pp. 1532–1543. https://doi.org/10.3115/v1/d14-1162.
80. Arora, S., Liang, Y., & Ma, T. (2017). A simple but tough-to-beat baseline for sentence embeddings. In *5th international conference on learning representations, ICLR 2017—Conference track proceedings*. Retrieved from https://github.com/PrincetonML/SIF.
81. Rücklé, A., Eger, S., Peyrard, M., & Gurevych, I. (2018). *Concatenated power mean word embeddings as universal cross-lingual sentence representations*. ArXiv. Retrieved from http://arxiv.org/abs/1803.01400.
82. Mou, L., Meng, Z., Yan, R., Li, G., Xu, Y., Zhang, L., & Jin, Z. (2016). How transferable are neural networks in NLP applications? In *Proceedings of the 2016 conference on empirical methods in natural language processing*, pp. 479–489. https://doi.org/10.18653/v1/D16-1046.
83. Kudo, T. (2018). Subword regularization: Improving neural network translation models with multiple subword candidates. In *Proceedings of the 56th annual meeting of the association for computational linguistics* (Volume 1: Long Papers), pp. 66–75. https://doi.org/10.18653/v1/P18-1007.
84. Sennrich, R., Haddow, B., & Birch, A. (2016). Neural machine translation of rare words with subword units. In *Proceedings of the 54th annual meeting of the association for computational linguistics* (Volume 1: Long Papers), 3, pp. 1715–1725. https://doi.org/10.18653/v1/P16-1162.
85. Merity, S., Keskar, N. S., & Socher, R. (2018). Regularizing and optimizing LSTM language models. In *6th international conference on learning representations, ICLR 2018—Conference track proceedings*.
86. Howard, J., & Ruder, S. (2018). Universal language model fine-tuning for text classification. In *Proceedings of the 56th annual meeting of the association for computational linguistics* (Volume 1: Long Papers), pp. 328–339. https://doi.org/10.18653/v1/P18-1031.
87. Ferri, C., Hernández-Orallo, J., & Modroiu, R. (2009). An experimental comparison of performance measures for classification. *Pattern Recognition Letters, 30*(1), 27–38. https://doi.org/10.1016/j.patrec.2008.08.010
88. Rutowski, T., Shriberg, E., Harati, A., Lu, Y., Chlebek, P., & Oliveira, R. (2021). Cross-demographic portability of deep NLP-based depression models. In *2021 IEEE spoken language technology workshop (SLT)*.
89. Carey, M., Jones, K., Meadows, G., Sanson-Fisher, R., D'Este, C., Inder, K., Yoong, S. L., & Russell, G. (2014). Accuracy of general practitioner unassisted detection of depression. *Australian & New Zealand Journal of Psychiatry, 48*(6), 571–578. https://doi.org/10.1177/0004867413520047
90. Vermani, M., Marcus, M., & Katzman, M. A. (2011). Rates of detection of mood and anxiety disorders in primary care: A descriptive, cross-sectional study. *The Primary Care Companion for CNS Disorders, 13*(2). doi:https://doi.org/10.4088/PCC.10m01013.

TABS: Transformer Based Seizure Detection

Jonathan Pedoeem, Guy Bar Yosef, Shifra Abittan, and Sam Keene

1 Background

A seizure is a sudden electrical disturbance in the brain. Symptoms include loss of consciousness, jerking movements of the extremities, and uncontrollable changes in emotional state. There are many types of seizures ranging in severity, locality in the brain, and reason for occurring. The temporal duration of seizures also varies, most lasting from 20 s to 2 min. Epilepsy, the fourth most common neurological disease plaguing approximately 2.2 million people worldwide, is characterized by unexpected, recurrent seizures. Thus, seizures are an ailment with tremendous scope [1, 2].

Correctly identifying seizures is of paramount importance. Firstly, misdiagnosis can wreak havoc on a patient's physical and emotional wellbeing. Medication is often used to treat a seizure; however, there are no clear guidelines on dosage. A doctor will administer medication and slowly increase the dosage, until the seizure stops. Moreso, proper identification of seizures is critical to prevent overdosing a patient. Secondly, if a patient is declared epileptic, his or her driver's license is revoked. This is one example of how seizures not only physically harm a person's body, but severely infringe on lifestyle. Finally, if a seizure is not identified, it will

J. Pedoeem
The Cooper Union, Electrical Engineering '20, West Orange, NJ, USA

G. Bar Yosef (✉)
The Cooper Union, Electrical Engineering '20, Miami, FL, USA
e-mail: bar@cooper.edu

S. Abittan
The Cooper Union, Electrical Engineering '20, Woodmere, NY, USA

S. Keene
The Cooper Union, Harrington Park, NJ, USA

I. Obeid et al. (eds.), *Biomedical Sensing and Analysis*,
https://doi.org/10.1007/978-3-030-99383-2_4

go untreated. These are just three of the reasons why proper seizure identification is critical.

Electroencephalograms, or EEGs, are the primary means by which physicians diagnose brain-related illnesses such as epilepsy and seizures. An EEG is a tool for monitoring the brain's electrical activity. Electrodes are placed on a patient's scalp to record the electrical waves emanating from the brain. The configuration of electrode placement can vary. The most common configuration is the International 10/20 Classifying Seizures in EEG Data System. In this system, 21 electrodes are evenly distributed over the scalp. The distance between electrodes is either 10 or 20% of the total distance from front (nasion) to back (inion). The 10/20 system utilizes four anatomical landmarks for positioning: the point between the forehead and nose (nasion), the lowest point of the back of the skull (inion), and the preauricular areas anterior to the ears [3]. See Fig. 1.

Voltage is always recorded relative to a reference point. Therefore, the next design decision in assembling EEG electrodes is the reference used. Two common choices are generally utilized. The first is AR, Average Reference, whereby the average of all the electrodes is used as reference. This can be unstable, so another

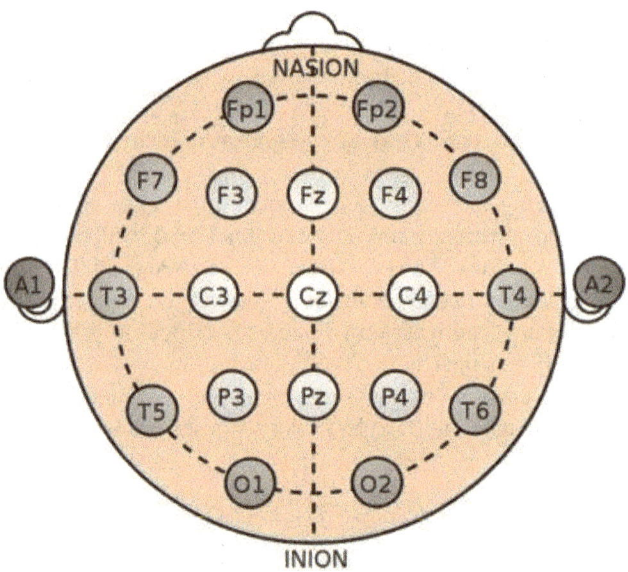

Fig. 1 The International 10/20 System for Placing EEG Electrodes on the Scalp. To record the electrical waves emanating from the brain, EEG electrodes are placed on the patient's scalp. The configuration of electrode placement can vary; this figure depicts the most commonly used system. In this configuration, the international 10/20 system, 21 electrodes are evenly distributed over the scalp. The distance between electrodes is either 10 or 20% of the total distance from front (nasion) to back (inion). The 10/20 system utilizes four anatomical landmarks for positioning: the point between the forehead and nose (nasion), the lowest point of the back of the skull (inion), and the preauricular areas anterior to the ears

popular choice is LE, Linked Ears Reference. In LE, a lead adapter links electrodes behind the left and right ears as a reference point. LE is believed to reduce artifacts [3].

Currently, a doctor must, either in real-time or subsequently, look through the EEG data to identify seizure occurrence. The doctor does not look at the raw EEG electrical signal. Instead, a montage is imposed on the data. A montage is a particular differencing scheme of the electrode channels in order to increase visibility of seizures and other abnormalities, while at the same time also reducing noise. The most common montage used is the bipolar montage. This montage is considered optimal for human detection of seizures [3].

Physician productivity and efficiency will increase significantly if a system could be built to automatically detect seizures. All current models that attempt this task have unacceptably high false positive rates. Therefore, hospitals do not utilize these automated systems.

Patients in hospitals are often hooked up to many different machines that must be monitored. The doctors and nurses do not want to be bothered by a seizure detection system that is constantly ringing for no reason. As such, only a system with a very low false positive rate would be useful.

2 Problem Statement

Properly identifying seizures from EEG data is a difficult problem. Even doctors with advanced training and a tremendous amount of experience, often disagree on the exact start and end times of a seizure. Seizures do not have a uniform waveform and can take on different shapes depending on the medication that the patient is taking. When a patient blinks, coughs or sleeps, the electrical signals collected by the EEG can either obscure or mimic a seizure.

Doctors spend hours every day reviewing EEG data in order to diagnose seizures. This is a tremendous drain on a doctor's time. Automating seizure detection could free doctors to spend more time at patient's bedsides, as well as care for more patients at a time. In addition, one doctor often reviews multiple patients' EEG files at a time. They stand in front of a computer as a couple of EEG montages fly across the screen. This is because for most of the file, no seizure is occuring. Because doctors review a few files at once, it is possible that they miss seizures.

Automating seizure detection is clearly important. However, in order for a detection model to be useful, it would need to have a very low false alarm rate. One doctor is often responsible for 12 patients hooked up to EEG machines. If each machine makes two false alarms in a 24 h period, the doctor would be required to come back to the hospital 24 times in one day. This model would be more of a burden than a help to the doctor. The current state-of-the-art machine learning seizure detection model has a false alarm rate of 7 per 24 h.

Therefore, we set out to build a machine learning seizure detection model with a very low false positive rate. While working on this project, Temple University teamed up with Neureka and created a competition to drive the research in this area forward. The scoring system in the competition placed a high importance on the false alarm rate, which aligned nicely with our goals.

3 Related Works

There have been several different attempts to algorithmically detect seizures in EEG data, spanning from signal processing to statistical analysis [4–12]. Deep learning has recently achieved state-of-the-art in image and pattern recognition [13, 14], and natural language processing [15–17] making it a great choice for this problem.

However, modern deep learning requires a tremendous amount of data to build reliable models. Historically, there was not enough labeled data available to apply these techniques to seizure detection. The Neural Engineering Data Consortium at Temple University set out to solve this data problem. They collected and compiled approximately 14 years of EEG data from patients at Temple Hospital and curated a corpus for research.

Version 1.5.1 of the corpus, released in March 2020, contains 642 subjects with a total of 1423 sessions [18]. 447 of these sessions contain seizures. There is a total of 922 h of data. Seizure events comprise about 63 h, or 6.8% of the annotated data. The data set also includes metadata, in the form of physician's notes. These notes include patient demographics and medication.

One great difficulty in building a seizure detection system, even if limitless amounts of data are available, is that seizures do not have a precisely defined waveform. Even while hand-labeling the data, the annotators often debate whether or not a particular signal qualifies as a seizure. Additionally, seizures often lack discrete start and stop times.

The current state-of-the-art model, developed by Temple University, achieves a false positive rate of 6 per 24 h with sensitivity of 30.83% and a specificity of 97.10% [19]. This model is made up of a time-distributed convolutional neural network (CNN) and a long short-term memory network [20] (LSTM) Fig. 2. They also applied pre-processing and post-processing stages, before and after the deep learning model.

The pre-processing stage takes the raw EEG files and extracts features from them, while keeping the EEG channels separate. To construct each feature data point, nine time samples were utilized, each 0.1 s long. The features extracted included linear frequency cepstral coefficients, differential energy terms and first and second derivative terms. The model input was a matrix of size 22 channels $\times$ 26 features. Each model input consisted of 210 time samples. Every time-sample was then passed through a convolutional neural network in a time distributed manner. These values were then recombined before being passed into a bidirectional LSTM.

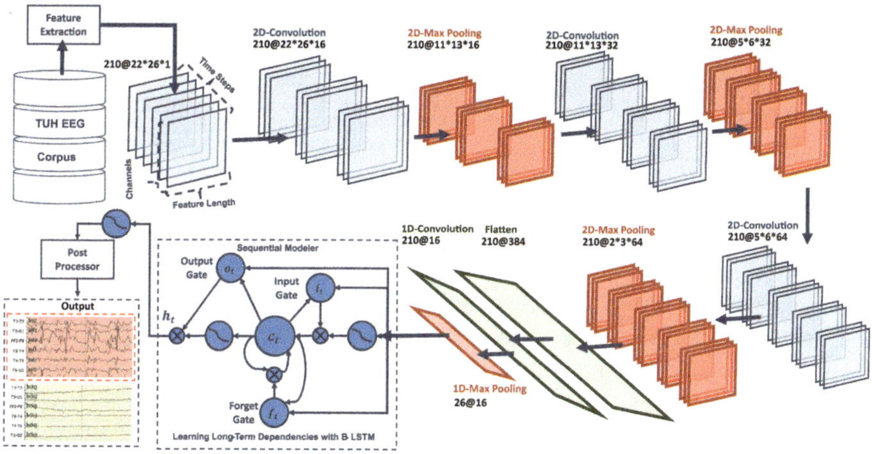

Fig. 2 The previous state-of-the-art model developed by Temple University. This model achieves a false positive rate of 6 per 24 h with sensitivity of 30.83% and a specificity of 97.10%. The model is made up of a time-distributed convolutional neural network (CNN) and a long short-term memory network (LSTM). Temple also applied pre-processing and post-processing stages, before and after the deep learning model. The pre-processing stage takes the raw EEG files and extracts features from them, while keeping the EEG channels separate. The model input was a matrix of size 22 channels × 26 features. Each model input consisted of 210 time samples. Every time-sample was then passed through a convolutional neural network in a time distributed manner. These values were then recombined before being passed into a bidirectional LSTM. LSTMs are helpful when working with sequential data. Finally, post-processing was applied, including a regression model, thresholding and filtering

Finally, post-processing was applied, including a regression model, thresholding and filtering.

The results of this model improved by two orders of magnitude from the post-processing alone. We believe that this suggests that the deep learning portion of this model is not accomplishing what it set out to do, with the majority of the detection falling on post-processing techniques. In our work, we hoped to leverage the deep learning model to its full capacity and eliminate as much of the pre and post processing as possible.

4 Motivation

Over the last several years, a team of researchers, based out of the Signal and Information Processing (ISIP) Lab at Temple University, have been working on automated seizure detection [21]. We began this project by familiarizing ourselves with the work that this group, led by Dr. Joseph Picone, has already accomplished. We met with the lab and learned about both their experiences and EEG data in particular, the primary source that they have been using in their research.

While getting introduced to seizure detection in EEG data and the work Temple University has already accomplished, the aspect that most intrigued us was the need for a model that will err on the side of caution when classifying a seizure; in other words, have a low false alarm rate. We felt that this requirement distinguished this project from anything we have dealt with before, and therefore we felt that a firm background in EEGs and the data they produce would be critical to our success.

In order to better understand what characteristics would be necessary for a good solution to EEG-based seizure detection, we first tasked ourselves with understanding why this is such a difficult problem. Because we did not have robust domain knowledge, as we are not neurologists that view EEG data on a daily basis, it was important for us to familiarize ourselves with the data through data exploration. We were keen to develop as much intuition as we could, believing that without doing so our contributions would be severely hindered. We wanted to avoid treating the data as a black box.

By doing this, we began appreciating the difficulty of the task. We scrutinized many EEG files using Temple University's visualization tool [22]. Although some seizure cases can be clearly recognized by an untrained observer such as ourselves, seizure and non-seizure labels may also be very difficult to discern. No matter how hard we tried to analyze the signal, there were seizure labels that were indistinguishable from background noise. By performing data exploration, we got to see firsthand that seizures and background noise can be nearly indiscernible. This is because EEGs are composed out of multiple voltage differences between the different electrode readings that are placed throughout a patient's head [19]. Technically speaking, the voltage difference used in EEGs leads to a very low signal-to-noise ratio (SNR).

Another interesting observation that we found while exploring the data was that even to the untrained eye one patient's EEG data could look very different from another patient's. Moreso, when referencing the accompanying doctor's notes, we learned that certain medications affect the brain waves, which causes very different looking EEG signals. Many medications suppress brain activity, causing the overall signal power to be much lower. A seizure, therefore, has many different waveforms, partially dependent on the particular medications that the patient may be taking.

After performing data exploration, we approached experts and tried to understand what heuristics they use in order to classify a seizure. We found that most successful professionals do not claim to have a set of heuristics, but rather a learnt intuition of what is and is not a seizure. We were surprised by the manner in which professionals scanned EEG files. They do not scrutinize each time sample, but instead go through most of the EEG in a cursory manner, almost as if skimming a book.

In hindsight, this preliminary data exploration phase of the project was a great way for us to become acquainted with EEG data in general, as well as the specific challenges inherent to seizure detection. After clarifying the problem at hand, we were tasked with choosing which machine learning techniques to leverage in our solution. We chose to focus on Deep Learning algorithms.

Deep learning methods solve optimization problems where gradient descent is utilized to optimize complicated functions with a large number of variables. Not only is this the subfield of machine learning that our team has the most expertise in, but it is also the class of functions that enabled Temple's laboratory to achieve their best results.

Deep Learning is an example of "Bottom Up" Artificial Intelligence (AI), as opposed to "Top Down" AI. "Bottom Up" AI describes an approach where the algorithm teaches itself how to make decisions. In a "Top Down" approach a researcher hard codes a series of hand-crafted heuristics. We posited that just as the professionals are using their own intuition to identify seizures, a machine should also be able to "learn" how to solve the problem, and as such a "Bottom Up" approach would be a great fit. This means that to replicate human performance, the model would have to learn an intuition of its own.

When deciding how to approach this project, our team decided to look specifically at the Deep Learning literature pertaining to Natural Language Processing (NLP). This is because there were several key similarities between an EEG channel and a paragraph of text. Firstly, both require context for understanding. In order for a reader to understand the meaning of a text, he or she can not look at an isolated letter or word—an entire line, and sometimes even paragraph, must be consumed. Similarly, one time sample from an EEG file does not provide enough information to identify whether the patient is currently suffering from a seizure. The surrounding time samples, or its context, is required. Secondly, both types of data have a sequential ordering. A sentence in English is read from left to right, while an EEG is read with increasing time. Thirdly, both EEG files and text can have variable lengths. Just as sentences are each a different length, EEG files are not of a fixed length either.

We felt that these similarities between language and EEG data strongly indicated that successful NLP models should also be successful in the EEG domain. However, we also identified some key differences between the two problem classes. Firstly, natural language is discrete, while an EEG is modeling a continuous variable (brain waves). Secondly, natural language has several delimiters, for example letters, words, sentences, paragraphs and chapters. Meanwhile, EEG's do not have any of these delineations, instead continuously transitioning from one value to the next.

At the time of our research, many of the state-of-the-art NLP models were using a Transformer-based architecture [23]. Due to both these recent successes and the fact that to our knowledge a Transformer had not yet been applied to the domain of EEG-based problems, we decided to utilize Transformers in our research. Transformers will be explored in a further section.

5 Data Pipeline

Over the course of our work we tried many different architecture types, experimenting with different deep learning elements and also tweaking hyperparameters such as their depth and width. We started our process with a hypothesis of what we intuitively thought made sense and then tried out several iterations of such a model with different hyperparameters to test not only if our intuition was correct, but also attempt to rule out bad hyperparameter choices as the reason a certain model architecture was not successful.

While we initially relied on our intuition and used it as a starting point for a hypothesis, we tried not to rely too heavily on it. Our intuition is only based on a few years of experience, so we tried to avoid letting it lead us into false biases of what we thought “should make sense.”

In an ideal setting, we would have an infinite set of computing resources. This would allow us to use a “spray and pray” approach, where we would be able to try any and every combination of architecture types, depths, widths and hyperparameters we could think of. Nevertheless, this was not our reality so we were left with trying to discern and rationalize which potential architecture type was the most promising to hedge our bets on.

In order to help facilitate our experimentation in this project, we developed a data pipeline that includes the following stages: pre-processing, training, validation, and evaluation. We built our pipeline using Pytorch [24], Facebook’s Machine Learning framework. The final two stages of our pipeline, validation and evaluation, also include a post-processing stage.

Although one of our goals was to avoid a pre-processing stage and to defer any signal enhancing techniques to our machine learning model, preliminary data exploration revealed that for our purposes at least some pre-processing was necessary.

As previously mentioned, we used the TUH EEG Corpus [18] to train our model. This corpus is the first collection of EEG data large enough to train robust deep learning models. As is the case with many datasets, however, it is not normalized. Specifically, different EEG files exhibited different channel combinations and were sampled at different sampling rates. This means that both the number of channels between files was different, as well as the channels themselves that were included. Additionally, each channel has multiple labels so that even if the same channel appears in different files, its name could be different in the two files.

We felt that these factors necessitated at least a minimal amount of pre-processing. We decided to compromise with our original goal and attempt to normalize the aforementioned aspects of the Corpus.

Firstly, we set out to resample the data to a uniform sampling rate. By running through the Corpus, we were able to compile sums of the number of files for each sampling rate. Our results are shown in Fig. 3.

We chose to uniformly resample all files in the Corpus to 250 Hz. Not only is it the obvious choice, being the smallest sampling rate in the Corpus, but we were cognizant of potential data bottlenecks we were going to encounter when loading the data into our model. We agreed that this was an effective compromise between retaining as much of the signal as possible, while still compressing the sheer amount of data we would need to compute.

We next set out to normalize the channel combinations by finding the overlapping set of channels among the files. Although all the files in the Corpus had at least 26 channels, the overlapping set among the entire corpus only consisted of 20 channels.

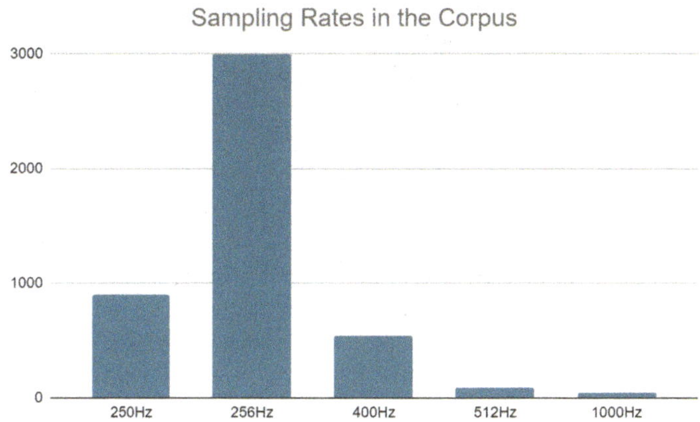

Fig. 3 The different sampling rates in the TUH EEG Corpus. The TUH EEG Corpus is the first collection of EEG data large enough to train robust deep learning models; however, it is not normalized—EEG files were sampled at different sampling rates. This figure is a compilation of the number of files present in the dataset, for each sampling rate. To normalize the data, we uniformly resampled the data to 250 Hz. This was an obvious choice, as it is the smallest sampling rate used in the Corpus. Additionally, this was an effective compromise between retaining as much of the signal as possible, while still compressing the sheer amount of data we would need to compute to avoid data bottlenecks when loading the data into our model

However we also decided to discard one of these, because many files had this channel zeroed out. Therefore we settled on a 19 channel set:

EEG FP1-REF	EEG F7-REF	EEG P3-REF	EEG T3-REF
EEG FP2-REF	EEG F8-REF	EEG P4-REF	EEG T4-REF
EEG F3-REF	EEG C3-REF	EEG O1-REF	EEG T5-REF
EEG F4-REF	EEG C4-REF	EEG O2-REF	EEG T6-REF
EEG FZ-REF	EEG CZ-REF	EEG PZ-REF	

Additionally, by using Temple's corpus [18] we were able to map and identify all the possible names used for each channel. Our end result on the input data was a 2D input matrix with 19 rows (one for each channel) and a column for each time stamp (with 250 columns per 1 s of time).

After analyzing the data we also found an undersampling of the majority class, with only 6.8% of the samples in the corpus being seizures. This is highly undesirable from a deep learning standpoint as it encourages the model to overfit and classify all inputs as non-seizure (what is sometimes referred to as the Accuracy Paradox [25]). Such a model would have an accuracy of 93.2% and would be useless. Given this problem we brainstormed several solutions, one of which was to use a different model like logistic regression which does not deal with this issue or to re-sample the training data to achieve a 50–50 split between seizure and non-seizure data. Some sources [26] strongly argue against re-sampling the data. However, as we were interested in using a deep learning model we nevertheless chose to go with this solution. The main argument against re-sampling is that the distribution between the training and real-world data will be different. However this was exactly our intention; we wanted the model to be more confident in its predictions of seizures.

The TUH EEG Corpus represented the ground truth in the form of a text annotation file which lists the start and end time for each background/seizure window. We converted this text file into a 1D binary output array with a 0 representing background noise and a 1 representing a seizure classification. This was done by generating an all 0 s array the same length as the resampled input matrix and then running through the annotations file and changing the ground truth from a 0 to a 1 during the 'seizure' labeled windows (multiplying start and end times by 250, the uniform sampling frequency we used).

Finally, we utilized Python's Pickle library [27] to convert the data into a binary format for more efficient processing. Each pickle file included:

- A 2D matrix of input data, with the rows representing channels and the columns representing time samples.
- A 1D array of channel labels (length 19).
- A 1D binary array of output data, with a 0 representing background noise and a 1 representing a seizure.
- A string that contains the doctor's notes corresponding with the current patient. While this was not actually used, we hoped to leverage NLP techniques on this string to better improve our model. While we were not able to perform any data visualizations on the data or confirm its usefulness, we hypothesize that the doctor's notes section contains a treasure trove of relevant data. One hypothetical example of this would be the medication that a patient is prescribed: it is very possible that certain medications alter the form that seizures exhibit in a typical EEG file, and that utilizing this information would improve a deep learning model significantly.

With our data preprocessed, we moved on to designing a flexible data loader that could be used in the training, validation, and evaluation stages by our machine learning models. We built our custom data loader by deriving from the *torch.utils.data.Dataset* class. Our initial implementation randomly sampled EEG data without taking into consideration which EEG file each sample belongs to. We did this because it allows the model to get its training data in the most random way possible, leading to a more robust model. However when we conducted empirical tests on our training stage, we noticed it was bottlenecked by I/O, with the data loader spending most of its time loading EEG files in and out of memory.

Our compromise was for the data loader to keep in memory a certain amount of files and sample data from these files only, until a percentage threshold is reached from each file. When a file's percentage threshold is reached, for example when 25% of the file was sampled, then that file would be swapped for a new one. While providing data that is less randomized to the model, it turned out to be more than an order of magnitude faster than our original brute-force data loader implementation.

Finally, we also designed data loaders to be able to input the data sequentially, for validation and testing purposes.

We trained our model in epochs of size 1,000,000. At the end of each epoch, we would calculate the training accuracy and checkpoint the model if we got a new best score. Additionally, every 5 epochs we would validate our model on a validation set kept separate from the training set. We then calculated the validation accuracy, sensitivity, specificity, and loss, and persisted a checkpoint of the all-time-best of each. Our checkpoint names included the hyperparameters used in the model that was being trained, allowing us to test out different hyper-parameters and easily save/load checkpoints based on them, as well as training and validation accuracy, sensitivity, and specificity values.

To increase our model's robustness, we used a data-focused regularization technique called mixup [28]. Mixup is a technique in which two pairs of training samples and truth values are taken and combined into one using a convex combination. This allows our truth value to change from a binary {0,1} (background or seizure) to the range [0,1]. We intended this to discourage our model from overfitting. The coefficient for the convex combination we used was taken from a beta distribution with its alpha parameter set to 0.6. This essentially kept beta around 0 or 1.

After our model was trained, we would test its efficacy on a separate evaluation set. We built a model agnostic script that accepts any model and associated checkpoint, running the post-processing scripts on the model outputs and finally scoring the result using Temple University's scoring script.

Due to both the practical importance of keeping the false alarm rate low and the large penalty attributed to it in the Neurika 2020 challenge, we experimented with several different post-processing heuristics including thresholding, vote-based smoothing, moving averages, and smoothing polynomial filters.

The first iteration of post-processing included a simple threshold followed by a vote-based smoothing system. The threshold converted the data from floating-point values to boolean seizure/background labels. For the vote-based smoothing system, we used a parameterized window size. Then, the middle value in the window was set to the most common classification within that window. Both the threshold value and window size were selected via quantitative experimentation. This post-processing technique improved our results by an order of magnitude.

After more experimentation, we found that if we smoothed the model outputs *prior* to applying the thresholding, our results improved even more. This intuitively makes sense because by smoothing the output before thresholding, a lot of the false positive jitter and oscillation in the output is eliminated. Then, the thresholding function can more accurately label each timestep.

For the pre-threshold smoothing task, we tested two types of low-pass filters: (1) moving-average and (2) Savitzky-Golay filter [29]. The Savitzky-Golay filter is a generalized moving average filter; it smoothens data by locally fitting polynomials of a specified order to it. After experimentation, we found that the Savitzky-Golay filter worked better than the moving-average, specifically with a polynomial of order 18. The dramatic improvement gained by our post-processing methods can be seen in Fig. 4.

Our finalized post-processing pipeline consisted of the Savitzky-Golay filter followed by a thresholding vote filter. Although not tested due to time constraints, we hoped to experiment with penalization when the model changes its prediction from one time sample to the next during the training stage.

After post-processing the model outputs, we were ready to score our results. Evaluating seizure detection models is not a trivial task. This is because the ground truth and predicted labels identify temporal events that span over many time steps; there is not a clear-cut answer as to how to consider and enumerate errors. Our problem is one of binary classification: seizure or background. All two-class problems have four possible types of errors: true positives, true negatives, false positives and false negatives. A true positive (TP) is when a seizure is properly identified as such by the model. A true negative (TN) is when a background label is properly identified by the model. A false positive (FP) is when a background label is identified as a seizure, and a false negative (FN) is when a seizure is identified as a background label. Based on these 4 definitions it is common to define the *Sensitivity* of a set of results as $\frac{TP}{TP+FN}$, and the *Specificity* as $\frac{TN}{TN+FP}$.

As defined by the Neureka 2020 Challenge, the "worst" type of error in seizure detection is a false positive and is heavily penalized in their scoring metric. This decision has practical roots, because when an automated seizure-detection technology is being used by a doctor or a health-care professional, many false positives will waste the medical personnel's time—exactly what the models set

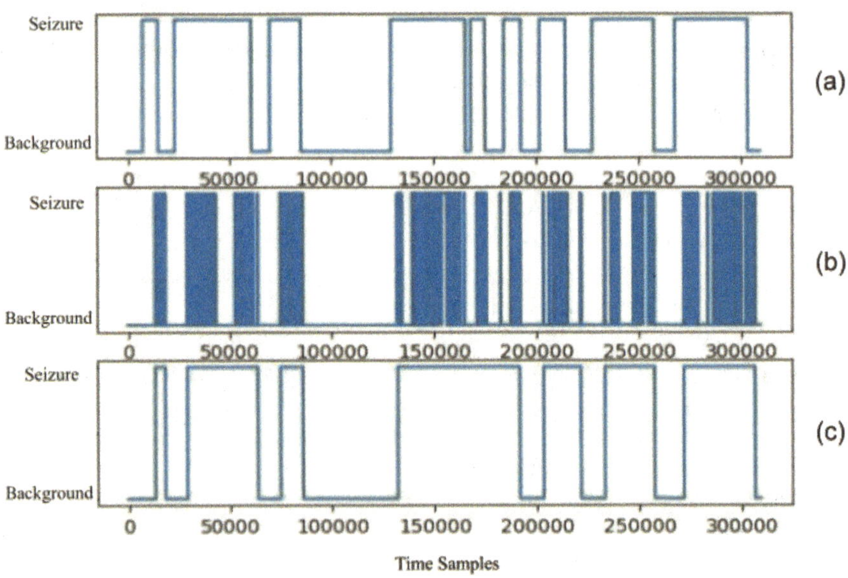

Fig. 4 The Effects of our Post-Processing. (**a**) Ground truth signal (**b**) Raw model output prior to post-processing. A lot of oscillation is visible. (**c**) Model output after applying post-processing (smoothing and filtering). Oscillation is now gone

out to solve. Therefore, although we of course hoped to have as high a sensitivity as possible, the main aspect we paid attention to in regards to our model's output statistics was to reduce the false positives.

Additionally, counting the errors in a predicted sequence is not straightforward. Often, the seizures identified in the ground truth and the predicted sequence overlap. Based on different criteria there is an array of different evaluation metrics available to treat this. The two that we focused on are Any-Overlap Method (OVLP) and the Time-Aligned Event Scoring (TAES) [30].

OVLP is the metric we initially worked to optimize. This metric is term-based and not frame-based, meaning that each individual seizure event is what matters, rather than a comparison of the label at each individual time sample. In OVLP, a true positive is counted any time the hypothesis overlaps in any way with the ground truth seizure annotation. Accordingly, a false positive is attributed any time where a prediction does not overlap at all with a ground truth seizure. The length of a seizure event as well as how much or how little it overlaps with the ground truth is ignored in the scoring. As such OVLP is considered a relatively permissive scoring metric.

The other scoring metric we considered, TAES, was the metric used in the Neureka 2020 Challenge [31]. This metric considers the percentage of overlap between events in the ground truth and prediction sequences and uses it to weigh the error. The true positive count is the total duration of a detected seizure divided by the total duration of the ground truth seizure. The false negative score is the fraction of the time that the ground truth seizure was missed divided by the total duration of the ground truth seizure. The false positive score is the total duration of the incorrect seizure in the predicted sequence divided by the total amount of time this seizure was incorrect according to the ground truth annotation. Temple presents a full description for each type of metric in [30].

When comparing Temple University's state-of-the-art model [19] under OVLP versus TAES, it is clear that TAES is a significantly stricter metric. The model achieves 30.83% sensitivity and 6.75 false alarms per 24 h using OVLP, while only 12.83% sensitivity and 7.54 false alarms per 24 h with TAES. We saw a similar gap in our own model scores when comparing the two metrics.

6 Results

When we initially started work on this project, we focused on implementing our data pipeline and general infrastructure. As such, our initial models were used purely for testing purposes. We created a model that classified every output as a seizure, another that classified every input as a background, and third that would randomly classify either or, with a 50% probability.

Following this stage, we created several exploratory models using only fully connected and convolutional layers. This allowed us to continue testing the data pipeline, while also seeing how robust of a model we can achieve without the use of any recurrent layers. A table of our different preliminary models can be seen in Fig. 5.

In this initial stage we evaluated our model outputs on a time-sample basis, comparing each of our outputs with its corresponding ground truth. As described earlier, this direct 1-1 comparison is not how the literature typically evaluates a seizure detection model. Moreso, this exploratory evaluation was conducted on only a subset of the full validation set that was released with the Neureka 2020 Challenge. This preliminary evaluation technique was used because we did not have our post-processing stage ready for use early on in our model development, however in hindsight the speed-up achieved by getting early results was likely hindered by these results not being directly correlated with how the Neureka contest evaluates model outputs.

When we finished building out our post-processing stage we were able to get a better understanding of our models using the OVLP metric. Although this was not the metric that ended up getting chosen for the Neureka challenge, our decision was made before the contest was announced with the motivation being that [19] described it as the most popular choice in the neuroengineering community.

Including the post-processing stage into our pipeline allowed us to both scale and add complexity to our models in the form of a recurrent layer. Using the OVLP metric as our discriminator we eventually settled on two models, which we call *transformerModel6* and *transformerModel7*, which we used for the final evaluation. These two models are nearly identical and so we expect results between them to be very similar. A table listing our model experiments can be found below Fig. 6. Some points about the table in Fig. 6:

- The sensitivity, specificity, and false alarms per 24 h (FA/24 h) are reported for the OVLP metric.
- **Dataset column**
  - *contest—50-50*: The training dataset provided by the Neureka 2020 contest, after we have normalized the number of seizures such that there is roughly the same amount of seizures as non-seizures in the data.
  - *resampled*: The dataset was resampled to a uniform 250 Hz.
- **Smoothing column**
  - *5000-1 x2:* Refers to our smoothing function that sums the 5000 elements before a current time sample and 5000 elements after a current time sample and sets the output of the current time sample to a 'seizure' classification if the sums are both above the threshold of 1, otherwise to a 'background'. This very aggressive smoothing function was found to significantly improve our results.
  - *sg: ws:fileLen, poly:18 → threshold*: Refers to the Savitzky-Golay filter being used with the parameters set to:

Model Description	Highest Train Accuracy	Validation Accuracy
3 Fully Connected Layers (FC3)	86	74
FC3 + CNN	85	78
FC3_WIDE + CNN	76	85
FC3 + CNN3	88	68.9
FC2 + CNN3	90.9	72.3
FC2 + CNN3 (all the following have larger windows 300 samples)	92.7	70.5
FC2 + CNN3 bigger batch size	90.7	71.1
CNN + FC2 + CNN3 (collapse channel dimension early)	88.6	64.1
CNN + FC2 + CNN3 (larger kernels)	90.1	69.4
FC2 + CNN3 (larger kernels)	92.6	73.4
FC2 + CNN3 w/ dropout	90.4	73.8
FC2 + CNN3 w/ Batch Normalization	95.7	73.4
FC2 + CNN3 w/ bn & dropout	90.8	77.9
FC2 + CNN3 w/ bn & dropout & l2 reg (0.1) (= + REG)	90.8	79.2
FC2 + CNN3 w/ bn & dropout & l2 reg (0.01)	92.2	77.8

Fig. 5 Our preliminary models and their results. This table summarizes the exploratory models we created using only fully connected and convolutional layers. This allowed us to test the data pipeline that we built, while also determining how robust of a model we could achieve without the use of any recurrent layers. The model outputs were evaluated on a time-sample basis, comparing each of our outputs with its corresponding ground truth. This direct one-to-one comparison is not how the literature typically evaluates a seizure detection model. In addition, the exploratory evaluation was conducted on only a subset of the full validation set that was released with the Neureka 2020 Challenge. We used this evaluation technique, because we did not have our post-processing stage ready for use early on in our model development

FC2 + CNN3 w/ bn & dropout & l2 reg (0.5)	86.1	77.1
FC2 + CNN3 + REG with more context (predict on 300 context of 600)	90	68.3
FC2 + CNN3 + REG w/ more context and more files in memory	96.7	49.4
FC2 + CNN3 + REG w/ more context, files & bigger epoch	83.5	64.3
FC2 + CNN3 + REG + MIXUP (0.2)	92.3	83.8
FC2 + CNN3 + REG + MIXUP (0.4)	91.3	83.6
FC2 + CNN3 + REG + MIXUP (0.6)	89.9	84.8
Replicated TU Model (CNN4 + LSTM)	93.4	81.0

Fig. 5 (continued)

a window size the length of the file
A polynomial of degree 18.
After the data passes through the Savitzky-Golay filter, it gets thresholded.

Surprisingly, our best results were achieved with the non-resampled training set, achieving a sensitivity of 30% and a false positive rate of 26.9 per 24 h.

On the official contest test set we used 19 channels and scored a sensitivity of 9.03% and a FA per 24 h of 31.21, giving us a score of −76.50. This placed us ninth place out of 14 contestants in the Neureka 2020 competition. The first place winners achieved a score of 12.37% sensitivity and a FA per 24 h of 1.44.

These results also demonstrate that our model is not as accurate as Temple's. We attribute several reasons for this. The first was our choice to minimize the pre-processing as much as possible. We believe that the low signal-to-noise ratio (SNR) of seizures in EEGs makes it tough for deep learning models to learn a strong feedback signal and that signal boosting pre-processing techniques are particularly useful in such cases. Secondly, due to time and computational constraints we were not able to fully tune our hyper-parameters.

Although our results do not beat Temple's state-of-the-art model, they are comparable. As such we argue that traditional signal processing pre-processing techniques, such as signal-boosting and denoising, can be delegated to a deep learning model. Alongside this, we also encourage more research into deep learning architectures with low SNR data.

Model Description	Dataset	Checkpoint	Smoothing	Threshold	Sensitivity	Specificity	FA per 24 hours
Transformer Model 6	contest— 50-50	maxSensitivity	5000-1 x2	0.8	24.2	0.67	35131
Transformer Model 6	contest— 50-50	maxSensitivity	5000-1 x2	0.5	26	0.73	32073.6
Transformer Model 7	contest — 50-50	maxSensitivity	sg: ws:fileLen, poly:18 -> threshold	0.3	30.86	86.7	33.85
Transformer Model 7	contest — 50-50	maxSensitivity	sg: ws:fileLen, poly:18 -> threshold-> 500-1 -> 50-1	0.3	30.04	88.86	27.38
Transformer Model 7	contest — 50-50	maxSensitivity	sg: ws:fileLen, poly:18 -> threshold	0.2	47.61	70.21	88.61
Transformer Model 7	contest — 50-50	maxSensitivity	sg: ws:fileLen, poly:18 -> threshold-> 500-1 -> 50-1	0.2	47.61	74.28	69.92
Transformer Model 7	contest — 50-50	maxSensitivity	sg: ws:fileLen, poly:18 -> threshold-> 1000-1	0.3	30.04	89.02	26.93
Transformer Model 7	contest — 50-50	maxSensitivity	sg: ws:fileLen, poly:18 -> threshold -> 50-1	0.3	30.04	88.75	27.67
Transformer Model 7	contest — 50-50, resampled	maxSpecificit y	sg: ws:fileLen, poly:18 -> treshold -> 50-1	0.2	26	83.83	43.11
Transformer Model 7	contest — 50-50, resampled	maxSpecificit y	sg: ws:fileLen, poly:18 -> threshold -> 50-1	0.3	14.7	89.05	28.18

Fig. 6 Description of some more advanced models experiments and their results. We used the OVLP metric as a discriminator to select two models, which we call *transformerModel6* and *transformerModel7*. These two models are nearly identical, and so we expect results between them

7 TABS: Design Details

Our final model consisted of a stage of Convolutional Neural Networks (CNN), a Transformer Stage, another CNN stage, and a two layer dense network ending with cross entropy. Between each dense and CNN layer we had a ReLU [32]. We also used batch normalization [33] and dropout [34] as regularization techniques after the CNN stage and after each dense layer. These architectures and techniques will be expanded upon further on, and can be seen visually in Fig. 7.

The first CNN layer consisted of a 1D convolution with an input size of 19 channels and an output size of 50 channels, a kernel of size of 5 and a padding of 12. Following the 1D convolution we apply 1D batch normalization, dropout with probability 0.7 and finally pass the output through a ReLU layer.

This CNN layer allows us to create a latent representation of the channels and have the model learn contextual information around each time sample of the EEG. This was inspired by the modern software that neurologists use, in which certain combinations for EEG channels are taken to provide a more coherent representation of a time sample than if all the channels had been displayed beside one another. We hypothesized that the model would be able to learn the optimal combination of channels on its own using this CNN layer. To continue the analogy between EEG and NLP, this layer can be seen as learning a "word" vector representation for each time sample of the signal.

As the name suggests, a CNN is based on the mathematical operation of convolution. Convolution is operated on two functions. Mathematically, convolution is defined as:

$$(f * g)(t) := \int_{-\infty}^{\infty} f(\tau)\, g(t-\tau)\, d\tau$$

Fig. 6 (continued) to be very similar. The sensitivity, specificity, and false alarms per 24 h (FA/24 h) listed in the table are reported as measured by the OVLP metric. The dataset column includes two possible values: *contest—50-50 & resampled*. *Contest—50-50* refers to the training dataset provided by the Neureka 2020 contest, after we normalized the number of seizures so that there were roughly the same number of seizures and non-seizures in the data. *Resampled* means that the dataset used was resampled to a uniform 250 Hz. The smoothing column includes two possible values: *5000-1 x2* and *sg: ws:fileLen, poly:18 → threshold*. *5000-1 x2* refers to the smoothing function that sums the 5000 elements before and after a current time sample and sets the output of the current time sample to a 'seizure' classification if the sums are both above the threshold of 1, otherwise to a 'background.' This very aggressive smoothing function was found to significantly improve our results. *sg: ws:fileLen, poly:18 → threshold* refers to the Savitzky-Golay filter with the parameters: (1) a window size the length of the file, (2) polynomial of degree 18, (3) thresholding applied after the data passes through the filter. Surprisingly, our best results were achieved with the non-resampled training set, achieving a sensitivity of 30% and a false positive rate of 26.9 per 24 h

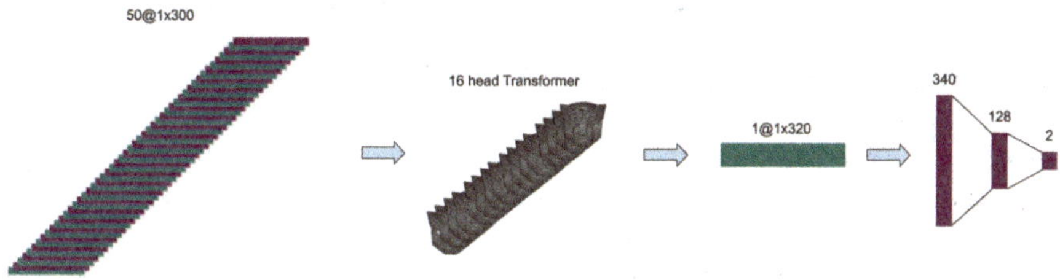

Fig. 7 Our Final Model Architecture. Our final model consisted of a stage of Convolutional Neural Networks (CNN), a Transformer Stage, another CNN stage, and lastly a two layer dense network ending with cross entropy. Between each dense and CNN layer we had a ReLU. We also used batch normalization and dropout as regularization techniques after the CNN stage and after each dense layer. The first CNN layer consisted of a 1D convolution with an input size of 19 channels and an output size of 50 channels, a kernel of size of 5 and a padding of 12. Following the 1D convolution we apply 1D batch normalization, dropout with probability 0.7 and finally pass the output through a ReLU layer. This CNN layer allows us to create a latent representation of the channels and have the model learn contextual information around each time sample of the EEG. Following the CNN layer, our model had a 16 head Transformer with a hidden dimension of 20. After the transformer stage we had the second CNN stage, where we used another 1D convolutional layer to form a linear combination of the 50 input channels, resulting in a single output channel. In this layer the kernel is of size 1, the dilation is of size 2, and the padding is of size 10. Similar to the first CNN layer, we pass this layer's output through batch normalization, dropout with probability 0.7, and finally a ReLU layer. The purpose of this set of CNNs was to combine all of the features that the model learned into a one-dimensional vector so that it could be passed through fully connected layers. The fully connected (FC) layers, making up the final stage of our model, were used to present our model's output in the correct dimensions required for evaluation. We wanted to project our model outputs down to two dimensions, so that we could use one dimension to describe seizures while the other labels background noise. The first FC layer goes from 340 to 128 dimensions, followed by batch normalization, a dropout of 0.7, and a Relu. The second and final FC layer takes the output dimension from 128 to 2

In English, to convolve means to roll together, which is exactly our purpose with the convolutional layers. To convolve two signals means to mix them by overlapping them and look at the result. More concretely, convolving a unit filter function with an input signal can be seen as a low pass filter, averaging out the signal locally. Visualizing convolution is a good way to get an intuition of why it is useful, and indeed in neural networks the goal of convolutions is often to provide spatial context.

In signal processing, convolving in the time domain is equivalent to multiplication in the frequency domain. As such, performing a convolution in the time domain can be interpreted as a scaling in the frequency domain.

This is useful in many different signal processing applications when one has a signal in hand and is only concerned about certain parts of it. It also allows the model to take into consideration context and filter out the unimportant parts of a signal. Instead of looking at a specific point in the signal, the model looks at the overlap within a window of points.

CNNs were first developed by Yann Lecun in order to recognize handwritten zip codes in 1989 [35]. He used back propagation to have his model learn the filter function directly from the data. His work set the stage for Deep Learning to break records in image processing, although it was not until Imagenet 2012 [36], 23 years later when this prophecy was completely fulfilled.

CNN is a slightly modified version of convolution where the learned filter function, or in the case of deep learning literature the 'kernel', is learned through gradient descent. In addition to performing convolution, a CNN layer usually consists of a pooling layer where neighboring values are combined, along with some form of non-linearity and often also dropout.

In Deep Learning the second signal is not flipped when convolving and the integral turns into a finite sum, as we are dealing with discrete signals. Otherwise the process is the same as mathematical convolution.

In our models we used a 1-dimensional convolutional layer, which acted upon the EEG signal's time dimension. With the first CNN layer we used the 19 common electrodes as channels and projected them out to 50 channels. Our intuition for this was to allow the model to learn different combinations of electrodes in addition to allowing it to just pass some of the electrodes through without combining it with other electrodes. If we were to project to less than 19 channels we would not have had this option. While this was our intuition, we have not confirmed if this is actually what the model learned.

The second convolutional layer in our model, following the transformer, took those 50 channels and merged them into 1 channel. This allowed us to prepare the latent layers to be passed through the final fully connected stage. Conceptually, it can be seen as the stage of the model where it picks the best latent features and projects them back down to a lower dimension.

Following the CNN layer our model had a 16 head Transformer with a hidden dimension of 20. Through empirical observation we found that increasing the hidden dimension layer beyond this caused our model to overfit.

Transformers are a Deep Learning model architecture introduced in 2017 in the hallmark paper *Attention is all you need* [23] by the team at Google Brain. Transformers were introduced as a model that can be parallelized more than recurrent models such as Long Short Term Memory (LSTM). This allows for the model to be trained more quickly, as it does not require the symbols to be introduced sequentially.

Transformers are based on Attention mechanisms. The novelty of a Transformer is that it uses a variation called Multi-Head Self-Attention. Attention is a function that allows an input sequence to be scaled based on importance. It is commonly understood as allowing the relevant parts of the input sequence to be *attended* to. Mathematically, attention (sometimes also clarified as 'scaled dot product attention') is defined as:

$$Attention\ (Q, K, V) = softmax\left(\frac{QK'}{\sqrt{d}}\right) V$$

Here Q is a query matrix, K is a key matrix, V is a value matrix, and d is the dimension of K. By taking the dot product of Q and K' we are loosely taking the cross-correlation between them. We then take the softmax of this dot product normalized by the square root of the dimension of K. This scaling is done so as to keep the values in a region where the softmax has a high gradient. Each row in the resulting matrix is a probability distribution which we then take the product of with the V matrix. All in all, attention can be thought of as attending to the parts of V that are the probabilistically most important, based on the Q and K matrices.

While the above paragraph describes attention, transformers use a variant called Multi-head self-attention. Self-attention means that all 3 inputs to the attention function are the values matrix (V). As such, it can be thought of as attending to the value matrix based on the value matrix.

Multi-head introduces multiple W projections that are learned through gradient descent.

$$Multihead\,(V, V, V) = Concat\ \ (head_1, head_2, \ldots, head_h)\ \ W^o$$

$$head_i = Attention\ \left(VW_i^a, VW_i^b, VW_i^c\right)$$

The addition of the W projection matrices allows for the model to essentially learn its own query and key matrices through gradient descent.

A Transformer (Fig. 8) consists of an encoder and decoder segment that is composed of multi-head attention units. The encoder consists of one multi-head attention unit followed by a fully connected layer while the decoder consists of two multi-head attention units followed by a fully connected layer. The second multi-head of the decoder takes as input for the query and key matrices the output of the encoder. In addition the decoder takes in outputs that are shifted to the right.

The input to the encoder is usually embeddings of symbols and not the symbols directly. In the NLP case this could be an embedding that is learned as part of an earlier part of the model or a pre learned word vector. In our case, it is the 50-dimensional latent representation of our 19 input channels.

Transformers have been a key part of the recent improvements in Natural Language Processing. Models such as Bert, GPT-2, GPT-3 [37–39], among others all use Transformers as the core part of their architecture. Often, it has been used in lieu of recurrent elements such as LSTMs [20]. It allows our model to take a large sequence of the signal in context, which we believed was very important for the seizure detection task. We therefore saw this as a great opportunity to try and experiment with them.

After the transformer stage we had the second CNN stage, where we used another 1D convolutional layer to form a linear combination of the 50 input channels, resulting in a single output channel. In this layer the kernel is of size 1, the dilation is of size 2, and the padding is of size 10. Similar to the first CNN layer, we pass this layer's output through batch normalization, dropout with probability 0.7, and finally a ReLU layer.

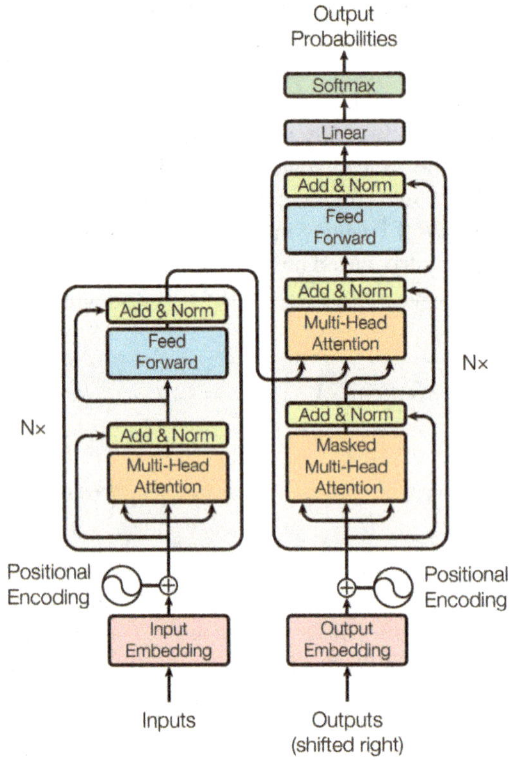

Fig. 8 Block Diagram of a Transformer. A transformer consists of an encoder and decoder segment that is composed of multi-head attention units. The encoder consists of one multi-head attention unit followed by a fully connected layer while the decoder consists of two multi-head attention units followed by a fully connected layer. The second multi-head of the decoder takes as input for the query and key matrices the output of the encoder. In addition, the decoder takes in outputs that are shifted to the right. The input to the encoder is usually embeddings of symbols and not the symbols directly. In the NLP case this could be an embedding that is learned as part of an earlier part of the model or a pre learned word vector. In our case, it is the 50-dimensional latent representation of our 19 input channels

This set of CNNs purpose was to combine all of the features that the model learned into a 1-dimensional vector which could then be passed on to fully connected layers.

The fully connected (FC) layers, making up the final stage of our model, are used to present our model's output in the correct dimensions required for evaluation. We wished to project our model outputs down to 2 dimensions, so that we can label one dimension as a seizure while the other as background noise. The first FC layer goes from 340 to 128 dimensions and is followed by batch normalization, a dropout of 0.7, and a ReLU, and the second and final FC layer takes the output dimension from 128 to 2.

Fully connected layers are one of the oldest neural network model architectures. A fully connected layer consists of only a matrix multiplication, yet it is almost always followed by some form of non-linearity to normalize the outputs and keep the model from overfitting.

In our model we used two back-to-back fully connected layers at the tail-end of our model. The first layer went from a width of 340 units to 128 units and the second layer went from 128 units to 2 units. We used a Rectified Linear Unit (ReLU) as our non-linear *activation function* after each FC layer.

A ReLU is defined as:

$$ReLU(x) = \text{Max}(x, 0)$$

Concretely, a ReLU zeros out all negative values. The benefit of having a non-linearity is to allow the model to learn non-linear projections of the data. If it were not for non-linearities, the best a FC model could do is create linear boundaries and there would be no use in having multiple layers, as they could all have been folded into a single matrix.

The ReLU is a favorite in the deep learning community for its simplicity and because of its empirically superior performance when compared to other activation functions. This is perhaps surprising, because the ReLU as defined above is not differentiable at zero. Nevertheless, the non-differentiability is solved by defining the derivative at the origin as either 0 or 1.

We also used dropout with a probability of 0.7 and batch normalization as regularization techniques in between these last two layers. These techniques were also used after each of our CNN layers. Regularization techniques are a common way to prevent deep learning models from overfitting on data.

Dropout is a technique in which with some probability each value in the projection matrix is zeroed out. One intuition is for there to be several different valid models that are contained within the main model. In our model we only experimented briefly with the dropout probability hyperparameter, but empirically found encouraging results when employing a very aggressive 70% dropout probability.

Batch Normalization [33] was introduced by Sergey Ioffe and Christian Szegedy in 2015 to prevent what they called internal covariate shift. What they observed was that due to randomness in the initialization of model parameters, the mean and variance of inputs to layers vary greatly. They claimed that this caused exploding and vanishing gradients. Exploding and vanishing gradients are the phenomena when the gradient is either really large, causing the model to ping-pong between outputs and unable to grow confident on any set of values (underfit), or the gradient is very small and the model learns almost nothing. Their solution, which they named *batch normalization*, is to normalize each training batch to have a mean of 0 and variance of 1. During model evaluation, the model would use a calculated shift from the training data to shift the test data as well.

After our FC layers projected our model's results into two dimensions, we used cross entropy as our loss function. This was done to create a probability distribution over the results and calculate a loss of how far our model was from the correct answer.

The loss function is used to come up with a final number that embodies how well our model is doing. Deep learning models then use a technique called back-propagation to 'learn' with respect to this loss value. Back-propagation takes the derivative of the model with respect to the loss and alters the model in the opposite direction of the gradient, which has the effect of minimizing it. In the case of cross entropy, a perfect model would have a loss of zero.

Cross entropy loss is defined as follows:

$$loss\ (x, class) = -\log\left(\frac{\exp(x\,[class])}{\sum_j \exp(x\,[j])}\right)$$

Where x is the output vector and class is the dimension of the correct class. What the cross entropy loss does is take the negative log likelihood of the softmax-ed model output. The softmax function transforms the output vector of the model into a probability distribution. It changes the output of the model into a confidence. The output of the softmax can be seen as the confidence that the model thinks this specific input belongs to a particular output class.

The desired outcome of the softmax function is to have a class with a value as close to 1 as possible, i.e. the model should be confident with its choice. As a sanity check, with a value close to 1, the output of the cross-entropy is, $log(1) = 0$, which aligns with our definition of a perfect model—if the model is correct we should not be updating it during back-propagation. For inputs in the range *(0,1]*, the logarithmic function is a strictly increasing function whose output is in the range *(−infinity, 0]*. As such, if the model is very wrong it will incur a high loss. Taking the negative of the log makes *(0,1]* go from *(infinity, 0]*, changing a maximization problem to a minimization problem, which was our desire.

8 TABS: Design Motivation

Our motivation is a combination of intuition and grid search. We started with several different assumptions of why CNNs and Transformers would be good models to use for this task. We then tried several different combinations and hyperparameter variations to see the highest accuracy we can achieve. We took careful notes of each iteration and compared results trial after trial to motivate our model changes. Figures 5 and 6 demonstrate part of this process.

9 Future Work

There are a few possible adjustments and additions that could improve the accuracy of Tables A general bottleneck in our development was training time, as we had access to only a limited number of GPUs. Due to a lack of time and resources, we were not able to fully explore these possibilities.

Firstly, initial values impact the stability of the model. By retraining the model many times, we can search the initial value space to find the most stable and fruitful set of values.

Secondly, hyperparameter tuning is in order. Proper hyperparameters in deep learning can often improve results significantly. Although we did do a significant amount of hyperparameter adjustment, there may be room for improvement in this area [40].

Thirdly, we hoped to experiment with penalization when the model changes its prediction from one time sample to the next during the training stage. That is, add a penalty to the model when the prediction switches from a seizure to a background and vise-versa. We hypothesize that this would decrease the amount of jitter in the model, leading to a smaller reliance on post-processing techniques.

Another small change we wished we had implemented was to run our post-processing and evaluation scripts during model validation as well, instead of only for model evaluation. We validated our model after every epoch, and kept the checkpoints with the best accuracy, sensitivity, and specificity values. As such, by not running our full post-processing pipeline during these validation steps we potentially chose less-than-optimal checkpoints.

Finally, we would have liked to incorporate data from the doctor's notes, such as patient medication, weight and gender. This information dictates the shape of the patient's brain waves and may help the model distinguish between seizures and background and could be used as a multi-modal approach [41]. For example, a patient who is already taking several medications may exhibit relatively subdued brain waves.

10 Conclusion

In this chapter we presented TABS, a novel model for EEG-based seizure detection. The design specification that was most important when developing TABS was achieving a very small false positive rate. The model architecture draws from cutting-edge, contemporary deep learning research: we built a hybrid architecture of convolutional layers, fully connected layers, and a transformer. Importantly, the only data preprocessing we use is grouping the data into uniform channels and resampling the time steps to a uniform sampling rate. This is noteworthy as it is significantly less preprocessing than what appears in Temple University's state-of-the-art model.

Our results are comparable to the SOTA and therefore suggest that much of the preprocessing used by Temple and others can be delegated to a more comprehensive deep learning model.

To view our code, please visit: github.com/guybaryosef/TABS-Transformer-Based-Seizure-Detection

Our conference paper can be found: isip.piconepress.com/conferences/ieee_spmb/2020/papers/l02_01.pdf

References

1. Seizures. Mayo Clinic. (n.d.) Retrieved from https://www.mayoclinic.org/.
2. Stafstrom, C. E., & Carmant, L. (2015). Seizures and epilepsy: An overview for neuroscientists. *Cold Spring Harbor Perspectives in Medicine, 5*(6), a022426. https://doi.org/10.1101/cshperspect.a022426
3. Ferrell, S., et al. (n.d.) *The Temple University Hospital EEG Corpus: Electrode Location and Channel Labels.*
4. Boashash, B. (2003). *Time-frequency signal analysis and processing: A comprehensive reference.*
5. Mera, M., López, D. M., Vargas, R., & Miño, M. (2018). Automatic detection of epileptic spike in EEGs of children using matched filter. In S. Wang, V. Yamamoto, J. Su, Y. Yang, E. Jones, L. Iasemidis, & T. Mitchell (Eds.), *Brain informatics* (pp. 392–402). Springer International Publishing.
6. Li, P., Wang, X., Li, F., Zhang, R., Ma, T., Peng, Y., Lei, X., Tian, Y., Guo, D., Liu, T., Yao, D., & Xu, P. (2014, November). Autoregressive model in the LP norm space for EEG analysis. *Journal of neuroscience methods, 240.*
7. Li, Y., Luo, M. L., & Li, K. (June 2016). A multiwavelet-based time-varying model identification approach for time-frequency analysis of EEG signals. *Neurocomputing, 193*(C), 106–114. https://doi.org/10.1016/j.neucom.2016.01.062
8. Rodríguez-Bermúdez, G., & García Laencina, P. (2015). Analysis of EEG signals using nonlinear dynamics and chaos: A review. *Applied Mathematics Information Sciences, 9*, 1–13.
9. Eichler, M., Dahlhaus, R., & Dueck, J. (2016). "*Graphical modeling for multivariate Hawkes processes with nonparametric link functions.*
10. Schad, A., Schindler, K., Schelter, B., Maiwald, T., Brandt, A., Timmer, J., & Schulze-Bonhage, A. (2008). Application of a multivariate seizure detection and prediction method to non-invasive and intracranial long-term EEG recordings. *Clinical Neurophysiology: Official Journal of the International Federation of Clinical Neurophysiology, 119*, 197–211.
11. Schindler, K., Wiest, R., Kollar, M., & Donati, F. (2002). EEG analysis with simulated neuronal cell models helps to detect pre-seizure changes. *Clinical Neurophysiology: Official Journal of the International Federation of Clinical Neurophysiology, 113*, 604–614.
12. Cherian, P., Vos, M., Swarte, R., Blok, J., Visser, G., Govaert, P., & Huffel, S. (2008). Automated neonatal seizure detection mimicking a human observer reading EEG. *Clinical Neurophysiology: Official Journal of the International Federation of Clinical Neurophysiology, 119*, 2447–2454.
13. Zbontar, J., Knoll, F., Sriram, A., Muckley, M. J., Bruno, M., Defazio, A., Parente, M., Geras, K. J., Katsnelson, J., Chandarana, H., Zhang, Z., Drozdzal, M., Romero, A., Rabbat, M., Vincent, P., Pinkerton, J., Wang, D., Yakubova, N., Owens, E., Zitnick, C. L., Recht, M., Sodickson, D. K., & Lui, Y. (2018). *fastmri: An open dataset and benchmarks for accelerated MRI.* CoRR. Retrieved from http://arxiv.org/abs/1811.08839.
14. Russakovsky, O., Deng, J., Su, H., Krause, J., Satheesh, S., Ma, S., Huang, Z., Karpathy, A., Khosla, A., Bernstein, M. S., Berg, A. C., & Li, F. (2014). *Imagenet large scale visual recognition challenge.* CoRR. Retrieved from http://arxiv.org/abs/1409.0575.
15. Devlin, J., Chang, M., Lee, K., & Toutanova, K. (2018). *BERT: Pre-training of deep bidirectional transformers for language understanding.* CoRR. Retrieved from http://arxiv.org/abs/1810.04805.
16. Wang, A., Singh, A., Michael, J., Hill, F., Levy, O., & Bowman, S. R. (2018). *GLUE: A multi-task benchmark and analysis platform for natural language understanding.* CoRR. Retrieved from http://arxiv.org/abs/1804.07461.

17. Brown, T. B., Mann, B., Ryder, N., Subbiah, M., Kaplan, J., Dhariwal, P., Neelakantan, A., Shyam, P., Sastry, G., Askell, A., Agarwal, S., Herbert-Voss, A., Krueger, G., Henighan, T., Child, R., Ramesh, A., Ziegler, D. M., Wu, J., et al. (2020). *Language models are few-shot learners.*
18. Obeid, I., & Picone, J. (2016). The Temple University Hospital EEG Data Corpus. *Frontiers in Neuroscience, 10*. https://doi.org/10.3389/fnins.2016.00196.
19. Golmohammadi, M., Shah, V., Obeid, I., & Picone, J. (2020). Deep learning approaches for automated seizure detection from scalp electroencephalograms. *Signal Processing in Medicine and Biology*, 235–276. https://doi.org/10.1007/978-3-030-36844-9_8.
20. Hochreiter, S., & Schmidhuber, J. (1997). Long short-term memory. *Neural Computation, 9*, 1735–80. https://doi.org/10.1162/neco.1997.9.8.1735.
21. Picone, J. (n.d.). Retrieved from https://www.isip.piconepress.com/projects/_index.shtml.
22. Van Beelen, T. (n.d.). EDFbrowser (Version 1.8.1) [Computer software]. Retrieved from https://www.teuniz.net/edfbrowser/.
23. Vaswani, A., Shazeer, N., Parmar, N., Uszkoreit, J., Jones, L., Gomez, A. N., et al. (2017, December 06). *Attention is all you need.* Retrieved from https://arxiv.org/abs/1706.03762.
24. Paszke, A., Gross, S., Massa, F., Lerer, A., Bradbury, J., Chanan, G., Killeen, T., Lin, Z., Gimelshein, N., Antiga, L., Desmaison, A., Köpf, A., Yang, E., DeVito, Z., Raison, M., Tejani, A., Chilamkurthy, S., Steiner, B., Fang, L., & Chintala, S. (2019). *PyTorch: An imperative style, high-performance deep learning library.*
25. Afonja, T. (2017, December 10). *Accuracy Paradox.* Retrieved from https://towardsdatascience.com/accuracy-paradox-897a69e2dd9b.
26. Harrell, F. (2020). *Classification Vs. Prediction.* Retrieved from https://www.fharrell.com/post/classification/.
27. Van Rossum, G. (2020). *The Python Library Reference, release 3.8.2.* Python Software Foundation.
28. Zhang, H., Cisse, M., Dauphin, Y. N., & Lopez-Paz, D. (2017). *mixup: Beyond Empirical Risk Minimization*, arXiv e-prints.
29. Savitzky, A., & Golay, M. J. (1964). Smoothing and differentiation of data by simplified least squares procedures. *Analytical Chemistry, 36*(8), 1627–1639. https://doi.org/10.1021/ac60214a047
30. Ziyabari, S., Shah, V., Golmohammadi, M., Obeid, I., & Picone, J. (2017). *Objective evaluation metrics for automatic classification of EEG events.* ArXiv, abs/1712.10107.
31. Neureka™ 2020 Epilepsy Challenge. (n.d.). Retrieved from https://neureka-challenge.com/.
32. Nair, V., & Hinton, G. E. (2010). *Rectified linear units improve restricted boltzmann machines.* ICML. Retrieved from https://www.cs.toronto.edu/~hinton/absps/reluICML.pdf.
33. Ioffe, S., & Szegedy, C. (2015, March 2). *Batch normalization: Accelerating deep network training by reducing internal covariate shift.* Retrieved from https://arxiv.org/abs/1502.03167.
34. Srivastava, N., Hinton, G., Krizhevsky, A., Sutskever, I., & Salakhutdinov, R. (2014). Dropout: A simple way to prevent neural networks from overfitting. *Journal of Machine Learning Research.* Retrieved from https://jmlr.org/papers/volume15/srivastava14a/srivastava14a.pdf.
35. Lecun, Y., Boser, B., Denker, J. S., Henderson, D., Howard, R. E., Hubbard, W., & Jackel, L. D. (1989). Backpropagation applied to handwritten zip code recognition. *Neural Computation, 1*(4), 541–551. https://doi.org/10.1162/neco.1989.1.4.541
36. Russakovsky, O., Deng, J., Su, H., Krause, J., Satheesh, S., Ma, S., Huang, Z., Karpathy, A., Khosla, A., Bernstein, M., Berg, A. C., & Fei-Fei, L. *ImageNet large scale visual recognition challenge.*
37. Devlin, J., Chang, M., Lee, K., & Toutanova, K. (2019, May 24). *BERT: Pre-training of deep bidirectional transformers for language understanding.* Retrieved from https://arxiv.org/abs/1810.04805.

38. Radford, A., Wu, J., Child, R., Luan, D., Amodei, D., & Sutskever, I. (2019). *Language models are unsupervised multitask learners*.
39. Language Models are Few-Shot Learners. (n.d.). Retrieved from https://papers.nips.cc/paper/2020/file/1457c0d6bfcb4967418bfb8ac142f64a-Paper.pdf.
40. J. Frankle and M. Carbin (2018). The lottery ticket hypothesis: Training pruned neural networks. CoRR.
41. X. Liu, P. He, W. Chen, and J. Gao (2019). Multi-task deep neural networks for natural language understanding. CoRR.

Automated Pacing Artifact Removal from Electrocardiograms

Christopher J. Harvey and Amit Noheria

Abbreviations

CRT	Cardiac resynchronization therapy
ECG	Electrocardiogram
LoG	Laplace of Gaussian
RMS	Root-mean-squared
$VTI_{QRS\text{-}3D}$	QRS 3D-voltage-time-integral

1 Introduction

The electrical activity from normal or abnormal cardiac muscle during cardiac excitation is recorded from the body surface in a standard fashion called 12-lead electrocardiogram (ECG). ECGs have been used to study the hearts in healthy and diseased patients for over a century. Cardiologists are adept in interpreting ECGs to diagnose cardiac structure and rhythm disorders. The main components of ECG, for every cardiac cycle, include the P wave from activation/depolarization of the upper chambers or atria, the QRS complex from depolarization of the main pumping chambers or ventricles, and the T wave from repolarization of ventricles. An example of a routine signal from one of the 12 ECG leads is shown in Fig. 1a.

C. J. Harvey (✉)
Electrical Engineering and Computer Science, University of Kansas, Lawrence, KS, USA

A. Noheria
Department of Cardiovascular Medicine, University of Kansas Medical Center, Kansas City, KS, USA

I. Obeid et al. (eds.), *Biomedical Sensing and Analysis*,
https://doi.org/10.1007/978-3-030-99383-2_5

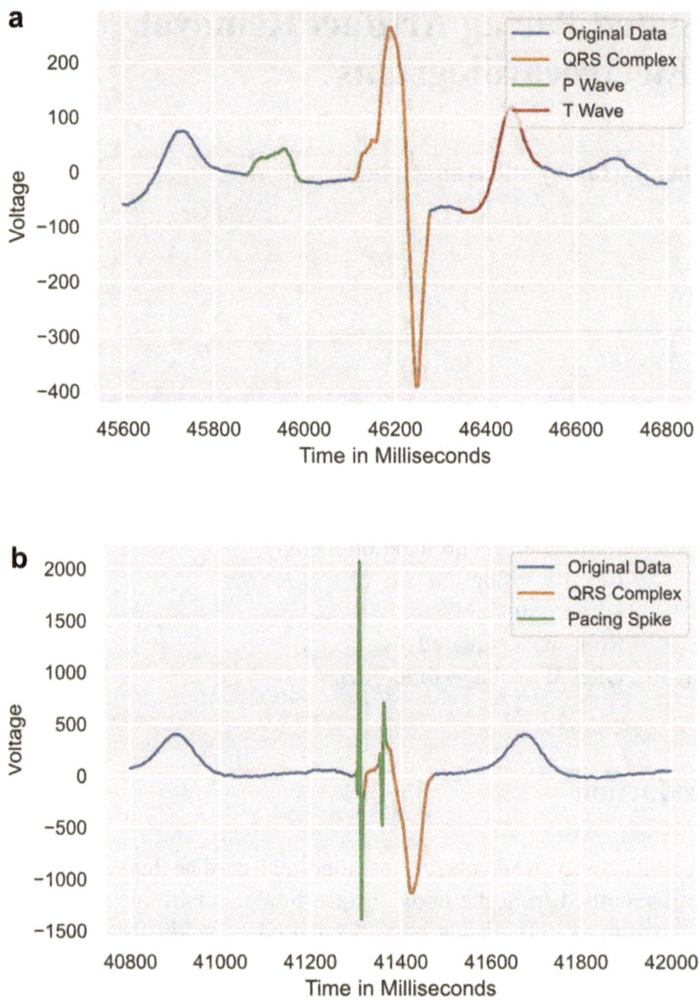

Fig. 1 (**a**) Example of non-paced routine ECG lead V6. The different parts of the ECG are highlighted in green (P wave), orange (QRS Complex), and red (T wave). The blue parts in between is the electrical baseline where no electrical activity is happening within the heart. (**b**) Example of ECG lead V6 in a patient with cardiac resynchronization therapy (CRT) pacemaker demonstrating pacing spike artifacts shown in green

Standard algorithms automatically quantify voltages and durations of the P wave, the QRS complex and the T wave [1].

The QRS complex captures the abnormal ventricular activation during intrinsic electrical disease, e.g. left bundle branch block, or ventricular pacing from a simple artificial pacemaker. This results in a prolonged QRS duration and increased QRS voltage, and sometimes results in heart failure [2]. The QRS 3D-voltage-time-integral ($VTI_{QRS\text{-}3D}$) or 3D QRS area is a novel summary measure of the electrical activity across the ventricles and has been validated as a superior measure of electrical dysfunction in patients with heart failure [2–4]. Sophisticated pacemaker systems called cardiac resynchronization therapy (CRT) can improve the ventricular activation with biventricular pacing, resulting in reductions in QRS duration and voltage [2, 5]. Recently, $VTI_{QRS\text{-}3D}$, after CRT is instituted, has been shown to provide improved prognostic information and may be clinically valuable in individually fine-tuning CRT system programming selections [3, 4].

Artificial pacemakers, including CRT, introduce large, short-duration, high-frequency artifacts, or "spikes", on the ECG recording when they deliver an electrical impulse to stimulate the heart. These large amplitude pacing spikes skew the ECG data [3]. The spikes that occur with atrial or ventricular pacing can often be ignored when performing signal analysis as the spike falls before the start of the signal of interest, P wave or QRS complex respectively. In these instances, the calculations would only be affected if performing analysis on the entire signal, rather than limiting analysis to the P wave or QRS complex, which are temporally consequent and distinct from the pacing spike. However, it is problematic if pacing spikes fall inside of the P wave or QRS complex as they skew any analysis on the data. This is especially relevant for CRT as there can be more than one temporally separated pacing spike generated within the QRS, with some likely to fall not at the onset but within the QRS complex itself (see example of biventricular paced ECG signal in Fig. 1b where the second pacing spike occurs within the QRS complex). Once a CRT pacemaker is active, such spikes can invalidate the automated calculation of various ECG parameters, e.g. $VTI_{QRS\text{-}3D}$. Thus, these outliers need to be removed from the ECG signal to automate meaningful and accurate calculations. This paper attempts to improve the measurement of post-CRT $VTI_{QRS\text{-}3D}$ by tackling the problem of pacing spikes. We will compare the performance of our described process with other traditional filtering methods for the measurement of $VTI_{QRS\text{-}3D}$ in CRT paced and non-paced ECGs.

There have been a number of different approaches to fix pacing spike artifacts [6–8]. The most common approach is low pass filtering [9]. Low pass filters retain the signal components below a certain frequency threshold and remove everything above the threshold. Correspondingly, high pass filters remove everything below a certain threshold. Band pass filters remove signal frequencies both above and below a certain band or a set of high and low thresholds. Band pass filtering works on ECG because the physiological ECG signal has a characteristic frequency range, and noise of higher or lower frequency can be filtered out. Most ECG systems therefore band pass the ECG recording at 0.05–1.5 Hz for high pass and 30–150 Hz for low pass. Additionally, alternating current electrical power supply noise (60 Hz in North and Central America, 50 Hz in most other parts of the world) is filtered out using a notch filter that eliminates a very narrow frequency range surrounding the local power supply frequency. Unfortunately, these standard filters do not do a very good job of filtering out pacing spikes in the ECG (as an example, the ECG in Fig. 1b is filtered 0.05–150 Hz with residual large pacing spikes).

To remove the pacing spikes, we need a new approach to find and eliminate the spikes in the signal. The approach we created builds off of Whitaker and Hayes's work on despiking artifacts from cosmic rays in Raman spectroscopic data [10]. We present our two-step approach to deal with spike outliers with (1) using modified Z-scores calculated from detrended data to locate and delete the large pacing spike outliers, if they exist, and replace the resulting gap using a hyperbolic cosine function, (2) followed by a median filter for lower-level artifacts. We customized the filter parameters for the ECG data with auto-adjustments to remove spikes without distorting the true physiological and non-paced ECG signals.

2 Data and Methods

2.1 Data Samples

The data for this paper was recorded on a Philips ECG machine with a standard 150 Hz low pass filter and a 0.05 Hz high pass filter. The sampling rate was 1000 Hz, meaning the temporal resolution of our data was one data point for every millisecond. The sample duration was 10 s. The Philips system generates an averaged beat from representative normal cardiac cycles in the 10 s recording. The averaged normal beat was used for all our calculations. The ECGs were recorded both before and after CRT. There was a large voltage artifact from the pacing spike in every CRT paced ECG. We included 90 patients who were diverse in age, race, sex, and height/weight. For each patient we included 16 ECG signals—12 standard leads (leads I, II, III, aVR, aVL, aVF, V1, V2, V3, V4, V5, V6), 3 spatial leads (X, Y, Z) reconstructed using Kors regression matrix [11], and a root-mean-squared (RMS) ECG signal made from the reconstructed X, Y, and Z signals. We thus had over 1400 ECG leads from 90 patients both without pacing and with CRT pacing. The RMS signal is used to obtain the QRS 3D-voltage-time-integral ($VTI_{QRS\text{-}3D}$).

2.2 Development of Our Filtering Approach

Outlier detection and removal: The first step of our approach was an outlier detection and removal process. Our process was built on work already done by *Whitaker and Hayes* on despiking Raman spectra [10]. Their approach involved creating an algorithm to detect outliers using a modified Z-score of once differenced, detrended data and then applying a simple moving average to remove outliers.

The Z-score in statistics describes how far from the mean a data point is by the number of standard deviations it is from the population mean. The standard Z-score is calculated as follows:

$$Z_i = (x_i - \mu)/\sigma \tag{1}$$

Where μ is the population mean, σ is the standard deviation, and x_i is any data point in the population. When using Z-scores for outlier detection, a standard threshold is 3.5 according to the American Society of Quality Control [12]. This value, however, may not be prudent for data signals that have long baseline periods of zero signal which exaggerates the Z-scores of the signals of interest. With ECG data, there are long periods of time between the T wave, the P wave, and the QRS complex where the heart has no electrical activity. These electrical baseline periods skew the population mean and make the QRS complex signal fall out of that 3.5 Z-score threshold. Furthermore, Z-scores are inconsistent as the mean and standard deviation of data are heavily influenced by large outliers. Whitaker and Hayes fixed this issue by using a modified Z-score approach which uses the median absolution deviation (MAD). The median value is much less impacted by outliers than the mean value. This makes it a better choice for outlier detection. The modified Z-score is defined by:

$$Z_i = 0.6745\left(x_i - \tilde{X}\right)/\mathrm{MAD} \tag{2}$$

Where $\tilde{X}$ is the population median, and MAD or median absolute deviation is the median of the absolute deviations from the population median.

$$\mathrm{MAD} = \mathrm{median}\left(\left|x_i - \tilde{X}\right|\right) \tag{3}$$

The use of a modified Z-score is recommended by the National Institute of Standards and Technology (NIST) as an outlier detection method [13]. However, a fixed cutoff threshold value may not be optimized for the precise characteristics of the artifact needing to be filtered. Furthermore, every heart is different and can have various structural or electrical diseases or scar tissue, and different spatial positioning relative to the body-surface that can drastically change the amplitude and relative frequencies of the QRS complex. Further, differences in heart rate affect the distribution of the modified Z-scores. This made ECG data unpredictable and impossible to have a set threshold to detect pacing spike artifacts for every ECG. Some ECGs need a modified Z-score threshold of 8 and others a threshold of 300 to accurately distinguish the pacing spike artifact from the physiological QRS complex signal.

To address this, we created an automatically adjusting threshold. This approach involved first calculating the modified Z-score distribution of the once differenced, detrended data. Next, we needed to identify the peak of the physiological signal within the QRS complex of the modified Z-score that was lower than a flexible criterion. Everything above this criterion should be spike outliers. The criterion depends on the type of data being introduced to the filter. If the data is non-paced, or does not have an outlier that is taller than the peak of the QRS complex, the

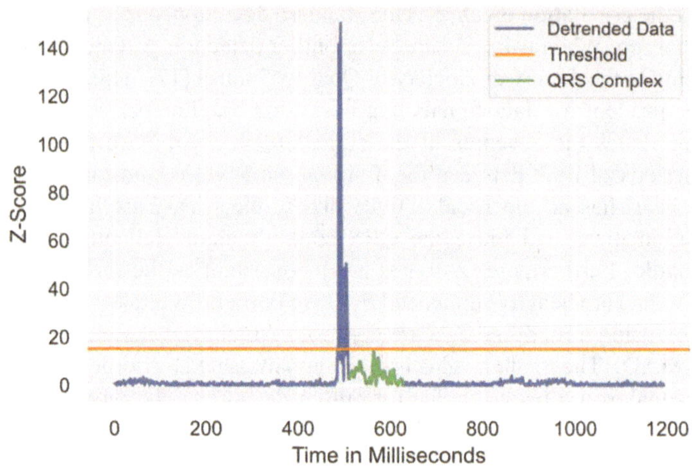

Fig. 2 Example of modified Z-scores of once differenced, detrended lead V4 data with automatic threshold detection just above non-outlier peak of QRS complex. The yellow line is the deletion threshold for outliers

threshold needs to be above the highest point in the modified Z-score distribution as anything above it will be identified as spike outliers. With paced ECGs that have an outlier taller than the peak of the QRS complex, we need the criterion to be just above the peak of the QRS complex. That way, the entire physiological signal would be spared and only the spike outliers would be identified.

The average maximum modified Z-score in non-paced ECGs is usually less than 70 and paced ECGs typically range 180–600 due to extreme outliers. If the largest value of the modified Z-score was at or above 150 we classified the ECG as "paced" as opposed to likely "non-paced". For ECGs classified as "paced", the criterion we selected was the value of the 98th percentile of the modified Z-score distribution, plus 40. This selection ensures the criterion to be greater than all the modified Z-scores from the physiological signal. The peak of the modified Z-score distribution that is below the criterion then identifies the highest physiological signal. We set the filter threshold to plus 1 above the peak within the QRS complex that was less than the criterion (Fig. 2). Everything above this threshold was thus identified as spike outliers.

We could not just set the filter threshold to the highest peak within the QRS complex, as pacing spike outliers can occur within the QRS complex itself. Instead, we used the criterion to find the non-outlier peak of the QRS complex. The selection choice of the 98th percentile in the criterion for "paced" ECGs was due to the nature of the outliers. They are typically the tallest datapoints in the dataset and are above this criterion whereas the entire physiological QRS signal falls below the criterion. We wanted a robust process that enabled automated identification of the pacing outliers but never included any data from the physiological QRS signal. The usual range of the peak of the modified Z-score of the physiological signal itself is

10–20 above the 98th percentile, though this can be a bit higher in ECGs with fast heart rates. We therefore selected the flat value to plus 40 to ensure the criterion was reliably above the peak modified Z-score of the physiological signal.

ECGs with a maximum modified Z-score of less than 150 were classified as "non-paced". Based on the typical distribution of modified Z-scores for non-paced ECGs, we selected the criterion to be the value of the 99.2th percentile of the data plus 55. We similarly set the threshold to plus one above the peak value within the QRS complex that is below the criterion. In the absence of outliers from pacing spikes, the 99.2th percentile (rather than the 98th percentile) as the cutoff brings the threshold closer to the peak physiological signal score. The flat value of plus 55 ensures that any non-paced ECG will not be affected by the filter.

The different distribution patterns of the modified Z-scores with and without the presence of pacing spike outliers is the reason why we do not have the same percentile and flat value cutoff for both paced and non-paced ECGs. If we were to use the 98th percentile for non-paced ECGs it would not work as efficiently as we would need a higher flat value especially for ECGs at faster heart rates. On the other hand, a higher percentile and larger flat value cutoff in paced ECGs would not effectively filter out all of the outliers. The 150 cutoff value to classify paced vs. non-paced does allow for some paced patients to be considered "non-paced", but the paced ECGs with max modified Z-score less than 150 tend to respond better to the 99.2th percentile method than the usual paced method. This allows us to be more robust in our overall process and allow some leeway to address any spike outliers in the "non-paced" group. In some cases, the margins between the pacing artifact and the physiological signal modified Z-scores can be quite small (e.g., modified Z-score of artifact is 72 and QRS peak is 69). In such ECG signals the outlier filtering step will only eliminate the tip of the spike artifact, and the remainder of the spike will be addressed by the second step median filter. The flat values and percentile values should be stable at 1000 Hz and 500 Hz ECGs. If the filter is used for other sampling rates or for other types of signal data, the user should look at the distribution of the Z-scores and adjust both the flat and percentile values accordingly.

We finally use a search method to find the peak of the non-outlier modified Z-score within the QRS complex that is below the criterion, ensuring that any extreme pacing spike outlier in the beginning of the QRS is not chosen. We initiate the search at the onset of the QRS complex and scan the QRS complex for the max modified Z-score. If we find a max modified Z-score that is above the criterion (percentile plus flat value), we redo the scan, this time initiating scanning 10 ms after the QRS onset. We repeat the process, each time starting the scan incrementally 10 ms further out from QRS onset through QRS offset. This process continues until we find a max modified Z-score that is below the criterion. We use a small value (5–10 ms) to iterate through the data as it helps to precisely avoid the pacing outliers when they occur in the beginning of the QRS complex and allow identification of a subsequent peak that fits our criterion. Once we find this non-outlier peak, we set the threshold that identifies pacing spike outliers to the value of the data point plus 1. This process is shown in Fig. 3.

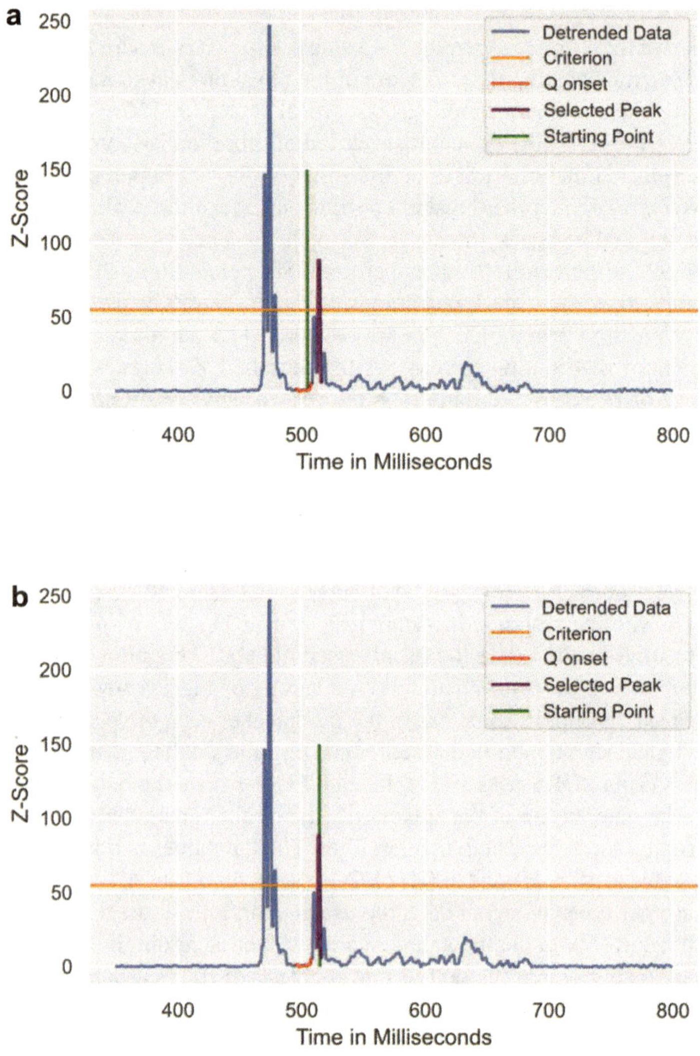

Fig. 3 (**a**) Demonstration of scanning process to identify non-outlier peak of QRS complex. Initial scan starts from QRS onset (red section) and then the max modified Z-score is found after the starting point (green line). The highest datapoint (max Z-score) within the QRS complex (purple line) from this initial scan is taller than the criterion (orange line), so the filter will reset and scan again further into the signal. (**b**) Demonstration of scanning process iteration. Subsequent scan(s) start from Q onset + 10 ms. The max modified Z-score (purple line) after the starting point is still above the criterion so the filter will reset and scan again further into the signal. (**c**) Demonstration of scanning process iteration. This time the max modified Z-score representing the physiological QRS signal (purple section) is found is below the criterion (orange line), and the threshold is set to plus one above this peak (yellow line). Everything above the threshold will then be deleted

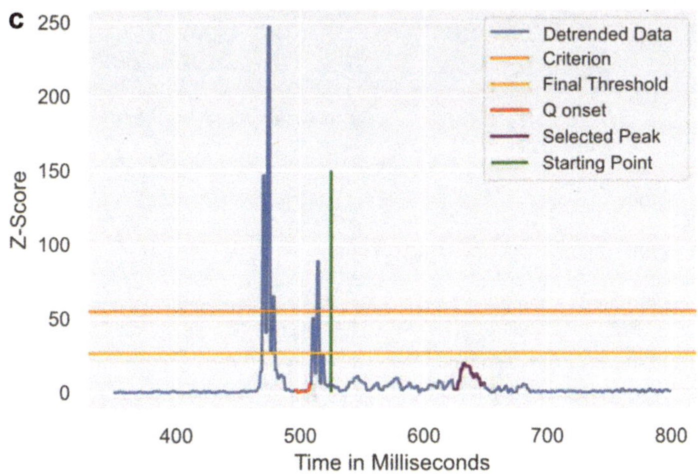

Fig. 3 (continued)

Once the spike outliers are identified, Whitaker and Hayes removed the spike by the neighbor interpolation method. Which is interpolating the mean of the values of the immediate data points before and after the spike that are below the threshold. This eliminates the spike outlier and smooths out the signal while introducing a negligible amount of noise to Raman spectra data. When this approach was done for ECG data, it did not work nearly as well because pacing spike outliers within QRS complexes have much higher Z-scores and longer duration of the artifact as compared to Raman spectra. The neighbor interpolation method diminished the outlier spikes without completely eliminating them and the spikes were still large enough to invalidate analyses on the data (see Fig. 4 at 400 ms). A median filter was applied after despiking to help with this problem. It achieved improved results but was still not completely satisfactory.

Our novel approach to this problem was to instead just simply delete all the data points above the threshold and fill in the remaining gap that is left behind with a hyperbolic cosine function (see Fig. 5 around 1700 ms) [14]. This is similar to the cubic spline interpolation method with a small difference in how the function fills in the gap. Deleting the spike outlier data completely removed any trace of the spike, and it is relatively easy to interpolate the presumed physiological signal from distant points. There are a number of ways to interpolate the missing data. We chose the hyperbolic cosine function to map the distance between the data points and create a slow building curve to connect them.

The hyperbolic cosine function is defined by

$$CosH(x) = \frac{1}{2}\left(e^{x}-e^{-x}\right) \tag{4}$$

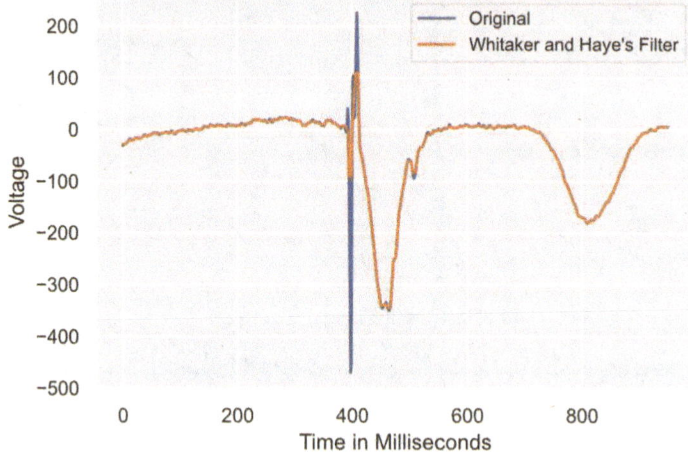

Fig. 4 Whitaker and Hayes algorithm on lead V4. Much of the outlier isn't removed because the filter uses moving averages

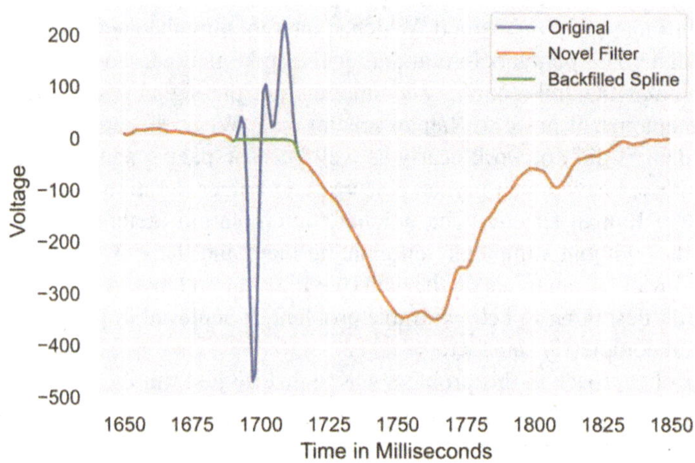

Fig. 5 Demonstration of novel filter on the same lead V4 from Fig. 4. The novel filter removes the data first and then interpolates which makes it much closer to the physiological signal

The whole function we used is described by four equations

$$\alpha = \frac{(y_2 - y_1)}{CosH\,(\tau * x_2) - CosH\,(\tau * x_1)} \tag{5}$$

$$\beta = y_1 - \alpha * CosH\,(\tau * x_1) \tag{6}$$

$$\gamma = Range\,(x_1, x_2, \varepsilon) \tag{7}$$

$$\delta = \alpha * CosH\,(\tau * \gamma) + \beta \tag{8}$$

Where y_2 and y_1 are the Y-axis coordinates and x_2 and x_1 are the X-axis coordinates of the two data points on either side of the deletion. τ is a small constant that determines how quickly the curve will build, where $\tau < 1$. We used a small constant (0.2) as we wanted our curve to slowly build up to better match traditional ECG signals. ε is a constant that determines the fidelity of the curve produced. We set ε to the distance between the two points on the X-axis. If it is not set to the distance between points it will result in the interpolation to have too much or too little data thereby impacting regression analysis and other techniques. The range function is a method that produces datapoints artificially so we can back fill the correct X-axis coordinates. It will produce ε number of datapoints starting from x_1 and ending at x_2.

The choice of the hyperbolic cosine spline, over a more traditional sine curve or polynomial spline, was due to the nature of the ECG data. ECG data typically ramps up voltage slowly, so polynomial curves are too aggressive to be natural on ECGs. The hyperbolic cosine curves are more gradual and follow the trend of the data much more closely compared to sine and polynomial curves. They do not need to have any data between the data points in order to operate. This makes them very fast but can be less accurate than more intensive methods. If the desired intermitted data points can be easily made from the type of data being used, then a polynomial spline is preferred. It proved quite difficult to create the intermitted data points for ECG data. So, we used the hyperbolic cosine function. Figure 5 shows an example of how our novel outlier filter works. It deletes all of the original information between the orange lines and backfills them with a hyperbolic cosine spline (green).

Second-step median filter: After extreme outlier deletion and interpolation, as a second step, a median filter is applied to eliminate any residual noise in the signal. This essentially acts as an intelligent band pass filter that filters out the high frequency outliers with dynamic precision and robustly cleans up low frequency noise. Median filtering is a non-linear digital filtering technique. It works by using a rolling median window across the data and replaces the data as it moves. The window size is determined based on the size of the signal being filtered as well as the size, shape, and amount of noise and outliers in the data. It is one of the simplest filtering methods and turned out to be most consistent among the multiple methods we tested as will be discussed subsequently. Based on the nature of ECG data and outliers, we used a window of 12 datapoints (12 ms) for the rolling median for this paper.

After filtering we added another check as a redundancy to ensure robustness of our process. Since the pacing spikes are very narrow, when they are deleted it should improve the accuracy of the QRS 3D-voltage-time-integral calculation but should not substantially change its value. If the change in voltage-time-integral is quite large, it would be likely that the physiological QRS complex was truncated by erroneous identification of the physiological signal as an outlier. We added a clause in the algorithm to revert the filtering process if the change in QRS voltage-time-integral between the original and filtered data was greater than 15% and flag the particular signal for manual assessment. The use of 15% as the cut off was decided by the average and standard deviation of change in the voltage-time-integral in all our paced ECG samples.

If the use of reconstructed spatial (X, Y, Z) or RMS ECG data is desired for analysis, filtering is more effective when done on the original 12 lead ECG data before doing any spatial reconstruction or the root-mean-square of the spatial data and was done in this way for this paper. This is because the outliers are not at the same location (X-axis) in each lead. These outliers are averaged when the X, Y, Z and especially the RMS is conducted, resulting in attenuation of the amplitude, and widening of the spike artifact, making it more difficult for our filter to eliminate and replace.

The step by step summary of our filtering algorithm is listed in Table 1.

Table 1 Stepwise summary of the novel algorithm to remove pacing spike outliers from ECG

Step	Action	Details
1.	*Outlier filter*	
(a)	Obtain modified Z-scores	Calculate the modified Z-scores of the once differenced, detrended data
(b)	Identify if paced or non-paced	If the max modified Z-score is ≥150 classify as 'paced' If the max modified Z-score is <150 classify as 'non-paced'
(c)	Set criterion	Criterion for 'paced' is 98th percentile of data + 40 Criterion for 'non-paced' is 99.2th percentile of data + 55
(d)	Identify peak non-outlier signal within QRS complex	Initiate at the beginning of the QRS complex with threshold value equal to 0 Look for the max modified Z-score value from starting point to end of QRS complex If the max value is less than criterion, set threshold value to +1 above that max value. If the max value is more than criterion, restart scanning process 5/10 ms further into QRS complex Repeat scanning steps until a threshold value has been found
(e)	Delete outlier data points	Delete all data points with a modified Z-score above the threshold value
(f)	Interpolation	Locate gaps left behind by deletion of outlier data points Fill in gaps using hyperbolic cosine spline interpolation
2.	*Median filter*	Apply median filter
3.	*Verify for unexpected truncation of physiological QRS complex*	If change in QRS voltage-time-integral is above 15%, revert changes and flag for manual review

We have subsequently applied our novel filtering process to a diverse set of over 10,000 non-paced and 10,000 paced ECG lead recordings for further validation. The results were consistent with what is presented in this paper.

2.3 Other Filtering Methods

Other methods that are typically used in signal processing, that we tried, include median filtering as already discussed, Hampel filtering, Laplace of Gaussian (LoG) filtering, and Butterworth filtering. There are other methods that we tried on our data that did not give as good of results compared to the methods discussed in this paper. We have omitted these other methods.

Hampel filter: Hampel filtering also uses MAD to detect outliers but it does not use Z-scores. It finds the rolling median and rolling MAD of the signal data and creates a threshold to target the outliers. The general equations used in Hampel filtering is as follows.

$$Rolling\_Median = Median\,(Rolling\,(x, k)) \tag{9}$$

$$Rolling\_MAD = MAD\,(Rolling\,(x, k)) \tag{10}$$

$$Threshold = L * \sigma * Rolling\_MAD \tag{11}$$

$$Difference = \mid x - Rolling\_Median \mid \tag{12}$$

$$Outliers = Difference > Threshold \tag{13}$$

Where x is the data signal. K is equal to the window size of the rolling functions. Because the window is before and after the center point, k is equal to 2 * window size +1. The size of k depends on the total length of the signal and how wide outliers typically are. σ is the number of standard deviations away we want to use for the function. For this paper we used a σ of 3 to target extreme outliers. L is the scale factor for Gaussian distributions (1.4826). We also used a k of 100 for both of the rolling windows. Hampel filtering is very good at targeting outliers and can be used with a very large signal to noise ratio. It tends to suffer when used on data with little to no noise though. This is more apparent in non-paced fast-heartbeat ECG data. The filter is more likely than others to treat the high frequency QRS complex as an outlier and remove it. The filter otherwise is very good. It does not have any parameters to tune other than window size and it is able to filter out very noisy environments.

Laplace of Gaussian filter: LoG filtering is a second derivative Laplacian convolution-based filter that uses Gaussian smoothing to deal with noise. Laplacian filtering is very sensitive to noise, so we use a Gaussian smoothing function to eliminate as much low-level noise as possible. For one dimensional signal data it is defined as such:

$$F(s) = \int_{0}^{\infty} f(t)e^{-st}dt \tag{14}$$

$$s = \alpha + i * \beta \tag{15}$$

$$Gaussian = e^{-\frac{1}{2}\left(\frac{k}{\sigma}\right)^2} \tag{16}$$

$$\omega = Gaussian\,(k, \sigma) \tag{17}$$

$$Z = F\left(x, \frac{\omega}{\sum \omega}\right) \tag{18}$$

Where F(s) is the Laplace transform function, which is a variant of the Fourier transform. We use the Laplace function to transform the Gaussian window and the signal data together into a single vector. S is the complex number frequency parameter with α and ß being real numbers. K is the window size. For this paper we used a window size of 12. σ is the number of standard deviations away we want to use for the function. x is the data point we are working with. ω is the Gaussian weighted window. Z is the filtered signal output.

LoG has an exponential decay function for the weights of the convolution. This means that the points closer to the center of the Gaussian window get more importance than points later on in the signal. As new data points enter into the window, the data is convolved together with the weights and filters the data. A weighted exponential decay function is used in the convolution to help deal with a lot of noise or large outliers. If only the moving average is taken, only a small amount of noise can be filtered out. Using the moving average also only works if there is a large amount of data. With limited data and lots of noise, something else is needed in order to filter out all the noise or outliers. A larger window size helps, but it can also lead to other problems if the signal changes drastically from the middle point of the window to the end of the window. For example, there is a big spike 90 data points away from the center and the window size is 100. If all the data before that spike is relatively flat, then the average for the whole signal will be skewed. So instead, it is better to use an exponential decay function based on the distance from the center of the window. It can also be the case that the future or past signal has rather different values not because of noise or outliers but just because the signal changes itself. Much like how the QRS complex skews an ECG signal. We would not normally want to take a large moving average with data such as ECG, but with the exponential decay function we can use larger windows. LoG also has the advantage that it does not have any parameters to tune or adjust. It is a filtering technique that works 'out of the box'. It is traditionally used for two-dimensional data such as images, but we wanted to try and use it for one dimensional signal data as well.

Butterworth bandpass filter: The Butterworth filter is widely used in signal processing. This is because the filter is maximally flat in the passband and approaches zero in the stopband. Meaning that it will filter out all data above or below the cutoff frequency range. The aggressiveness of the filter is based on the order. The higher the order the more quickly the stop band will tend towards zero (Fig. 6). A Butterworth bandpass filter transfer function with no filter gain is described by:

$$|Low(jw)| = \frac{1}{\sqrt{1 + \left(\frac{\omega}{\omega_c}\right)^{2n}}} \tag{19}$$

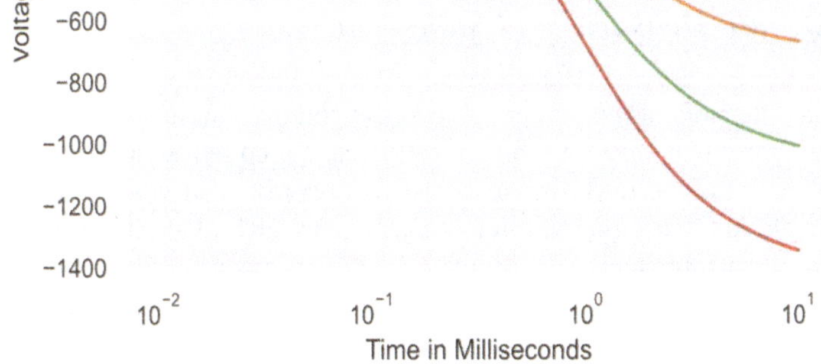

Fig. 6 Phase Bode plot comparing effect of order size on Butterworth filter

$$|High(jw)| = \frac{\omega^n}{\sqrt{1 + \omega^{2n}}} \tag{20}$$

Where ω is the angular frequency of the filter. ω_c is the cutoff frequency of the filter. n is the filter order. In the method we used, we did a forward and backward pass of the Butterworth digital filter. We had a frequency of 1000 Hz, an order of 3, and tried a cutoff frequency of 60, 90, 120, and 150 Hz.

All of these filter parameter selections have tradeoffs. Each selection is either good for paced or good for non-paced ECGs. The general tradeoff is a simple question. Do we want to better remove the outlier, or do we want to ensure the QRS complex is left unimpacted? The only filter that does not have this question applicable to it is the Hampel filter. The Hampel filter does well with large pacing spike outliers. It just fails to perform with a high standard with non-paced ECGs as it treats the QRS complex as an outlier. For median filtering, if we made the window larger for the rolling median to remove more of the outlier it would also start to flatten out the QRS complex. If we made the window smaller it would not distort the QRS complex, but it would also barely diminish the amplitude of the outlier. There is also the issue of the width of the outlier. If the outlier is wider than the window used in LoG, Median, Whitaker and Hayes, or Hampel filtering, the filters will either break or suffer heavily. So, we cannot use too small of a window because it will become ineffectual, but we also cannot use too big of a window or it will change the QRS complex. This tradeoff is also evident in filtering techniques that do not use rolling windows such as the Butterworth filter. A low cutoff frequency of 60 Hz will greatly diminish the outlier, but it will also change the fundamental structure of the QRS complex for both paced and non-paced ECGs. If a higher low cutoff frequency of 150 Hz is selected, the QRS complex remains untouched but so does the outlier, which can even be exaggerated. This tradeoff is the main problem that limits the traditional filtering methods for pacing spike removal. We developed the novel process described in this paper, as a solution to this problem.

2.4 Outcome Measures and Statistical Testing

We evaluated the area of the outlier spike as the voltage-time-integral encompassed above a straight line connecting the physiological signal before and after the spike artifact. A % reduction in the spike area was thus obtained when comparing the filtered signals to the original unfiltered signal. The QRS 3D-voltage-time-integral ($VTI_{QRS\text{-}3D}$) was obtained from the RMS of the reconstructed X, Y, Z leads obtained from the 12-lead ECG signals that were processed using the respective various filtering methods. We evaluated the impact of the various methods for filtering pacing spike artifacts on calculation of $VTI_{QRS\text{-}3D}$ as the absolute change in $VTI_{QRS\text{-}3D}$ in both CRT paced and non-paced ECGs. For this we used pairwise t-tests comparing the filtered versus unfiltered ECGs.

3 Results

We studied 90 ECGs with CRT pacing artifacts within the QRS, and 90 normal ECGs without pacing artifacts as controls. The same filter parameters were used for all tables and figures.

In the paced group, the unfiltered $VTI_{QRS\text{-}3D}$ was 67.9 ± 32.7 μVs and decreased with outlier filtering to 67.2 ± 32.5 μVs (p = 0.001). In the non-paced control group, the outlier filter did not affect $VTI_{QRS\text{-}3D}$ (both 41.8 ± 10.4, p = 0.7). With subsequent median filtering, the paced $VTI_{QRS\text{-}3D}$ slightly changed to 67.6 ± 32.5 ($p = 1 \times 10^{-9}$) and the control $VTI_{QRS\text{-}3D}$ to 41.4 ± 10.4 ($p = 2 \times 10^{-6}$). This indicates that the first step of outlier filtering only changes the paced ECGs and does not affect the non-paced ECGs. The second step median filtering does change both because of the nature of the filter but the overall change in area was negligible in both groups. The noise was smoothed out with only minor changes to the physiological signal.

Figure 7 shows how each step of the filter affects the data. The leads in the figure are the root-mean-square of our reconstructed spatial (X, Y, Z) ECG. The two examples are among the hardest paced and non-paced ECGs we found in our dataset to effectively filter using various filtering methods. We compare all of the filtering techniques on this data to show the differences between them using different filtering methods (Figs. 8, 9, 10, 11, 12, 13, 14, 15, and 16).

We can see in Fig. 7 that the novel filter removes a majority of the first main outlier but not the second spike that is within the QRS complex or the QRS complex itself. The outlier filter also does not change any of the non-paced control signal. This shows that this filter only targets outliers with dynamic precision. The second step median filter further smooths out both outliers in the paced ECG and the low-level noise before and after the QRS in the non-paced ECG. The median filter works well in this case as the major spike has already been removed making the outlier closer to the true signal. We can also see that the median filter barely changes the non-paced signal as the peak amplitude is trivially reduced and low-level noise is filtered out. This is the best result we have gotten on this data with batch filtering algorithmically and not selecting parameters individually for these cases. If we were to tune this filter for individual use, we could perfectly remove the outlier and leave the non-paced ECG unchanged. However, the idea is to have an automated filter that should be able to be applied on hundreds of thousands of ECGs without human intervention.

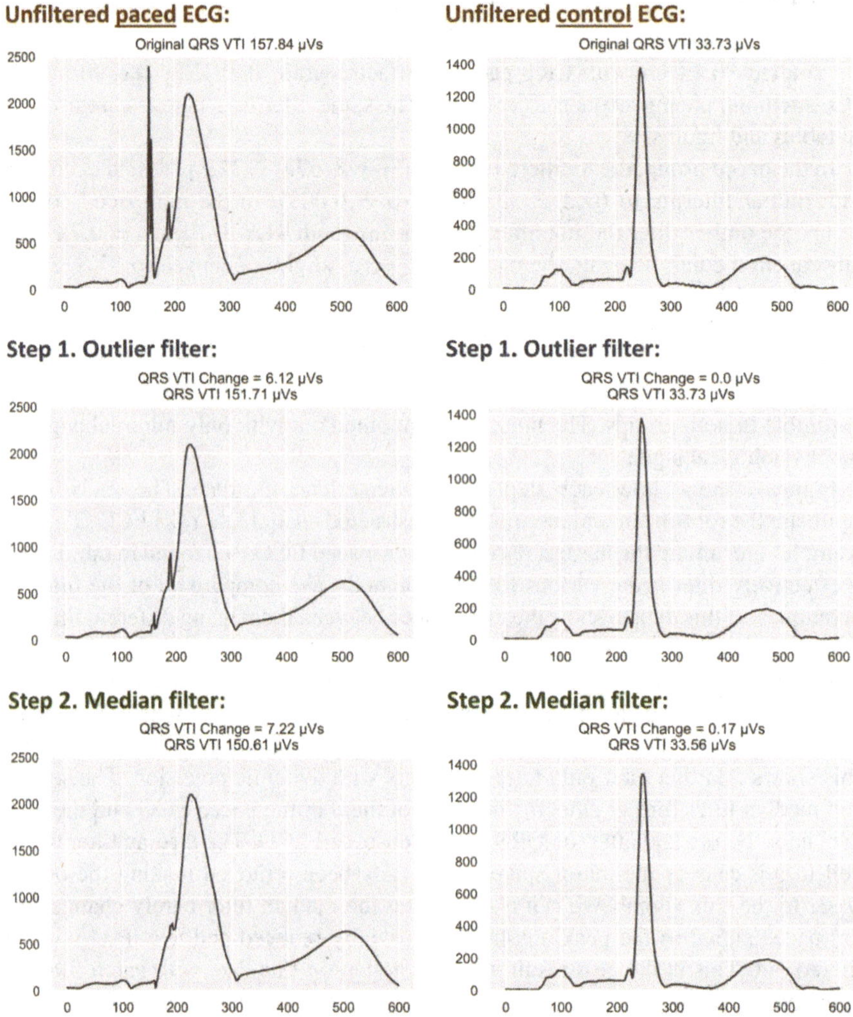

Fig. 7 Two examples of *novel two-step filter* on a cardiac resynchronization therapy (CRT) paced and a non-paced (control) RMS ECG signal. The novel filter successfully filters out the paced outliers while not augmenting the non-paced ECG

Compare this with Fig. 8 which is only the median filter applied. We can see that there is basically the same change to the control group. When we compare the paced ECG, it is a different story. The median filter only removes 1.32 μVs of the spike area compared to 7.22 μVs for our novel method. We can see that the removal of the major spike before median filtering in our filtering process makes a massive difference in the overall quality of filtering.

The Hampel filtering (Fig. 9) is second-best only to our novel method for paced ECGs, but too aggressive with non-paced ECGs. It has a 3.33 μVs reduction in area

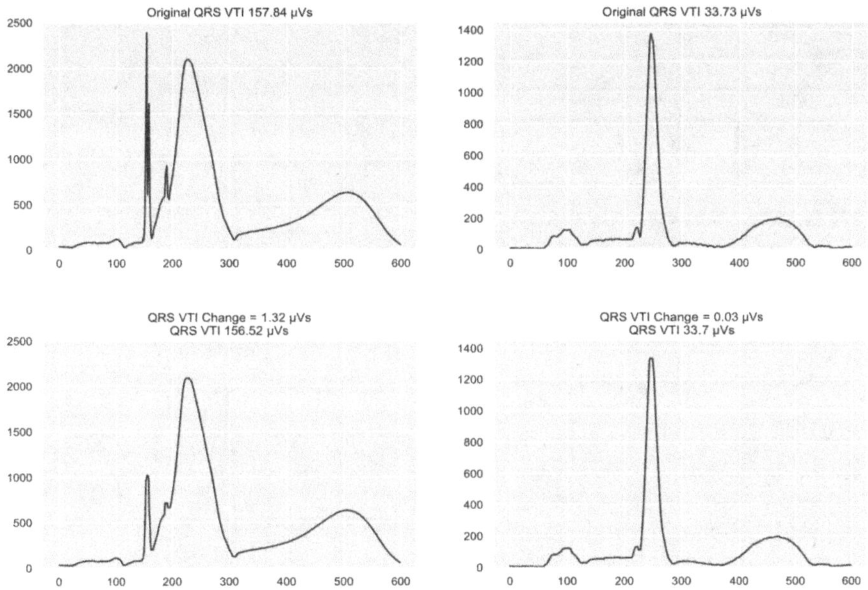

Fig. 8 Same two examples with *median filter* on a cardiac resynchronization therapy (CRT) paced and a non-paced (control) RMS ECG signal

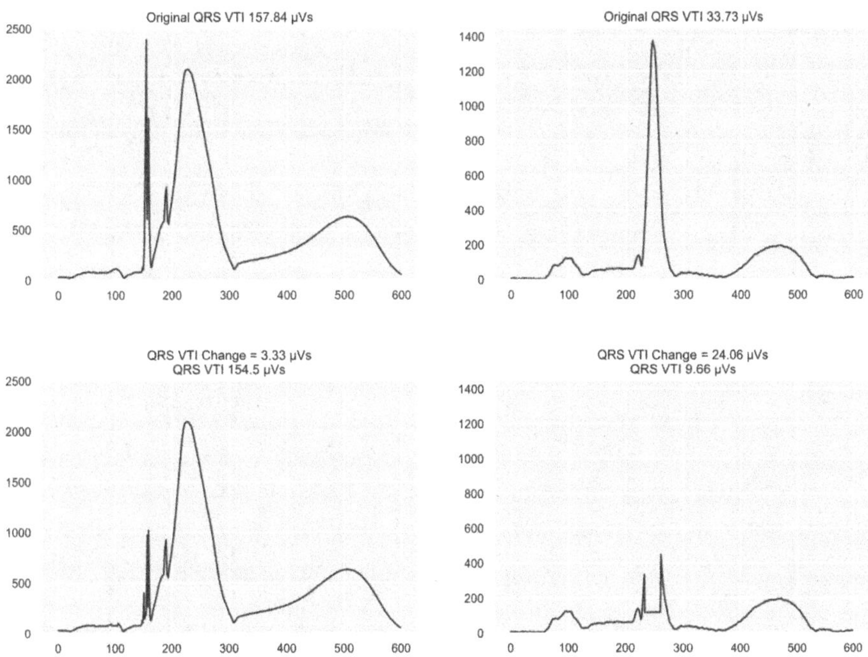

Fig. 9 Same two examples with *Hampel filter* on a cardiac resynchronization therapy (CRT) paced and a non-paced (control) RMS ECG signal

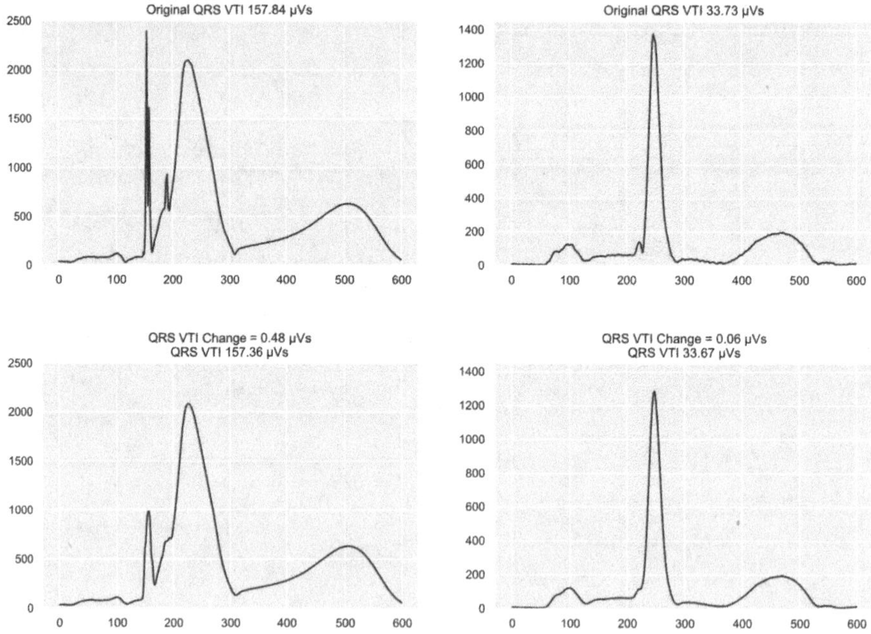

Fig. 10 Same two examples with *Laplace of Gaussian (LoG) filter* on a cardiac resynchronization therapy (CRT) paced and a non-paced (control) RMS ECG signal

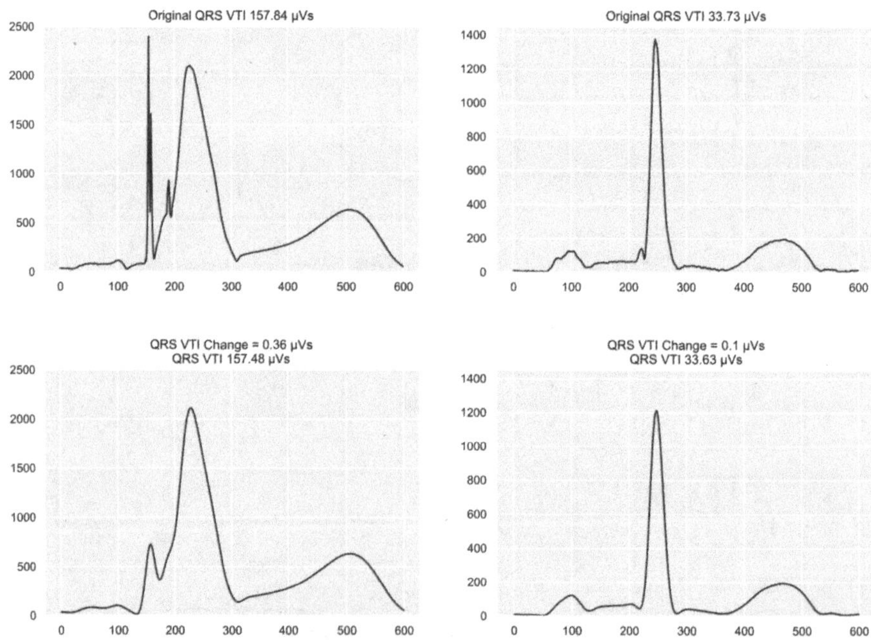

Fig. 11 Same two examples with *60 Hz Butterworth low pass filter* on a cardiac resynchronization therapy (CRT) paced and a non-paced (control) RMS ECG signal

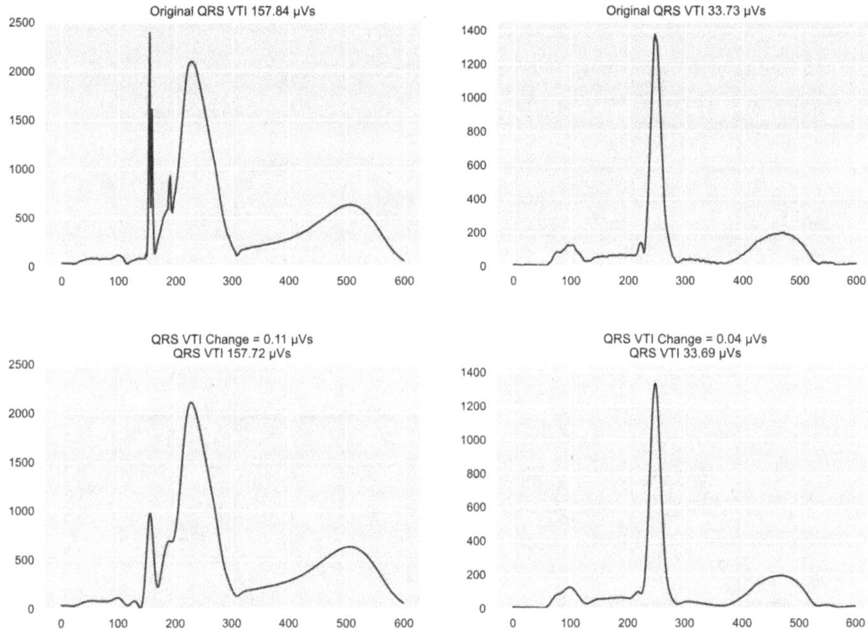

Fig. 12 Same two examples with *90 Hz Butterworth low pass filter* on a cardiac resynchronization therapy (CRT) paced and a non-paced (control) RMS ECG signal

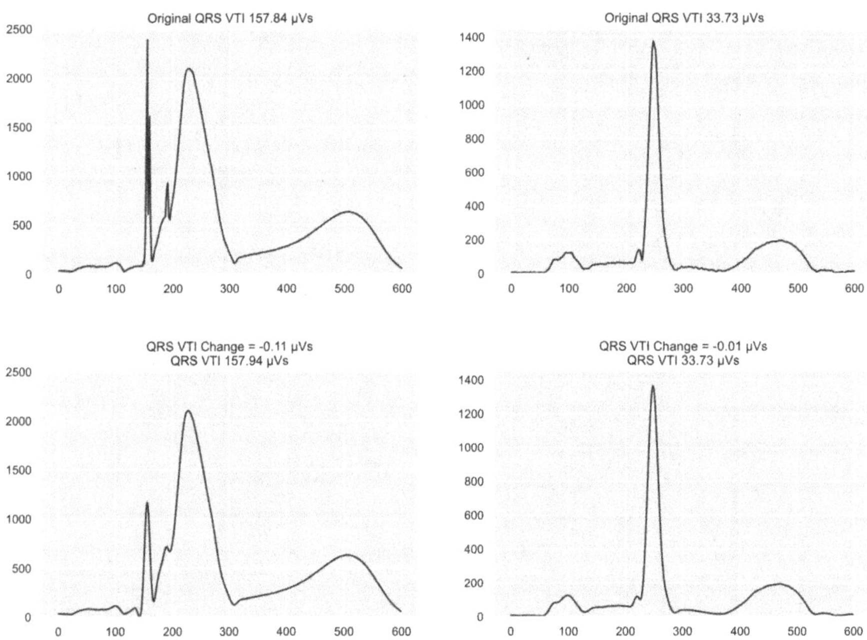

Fig. 13 Same two examples with *120 Hz Butterworth low pass filter* on a cardiac resynchronization therapy (CRT) paced and a non-paced (control) RMS ECG signal

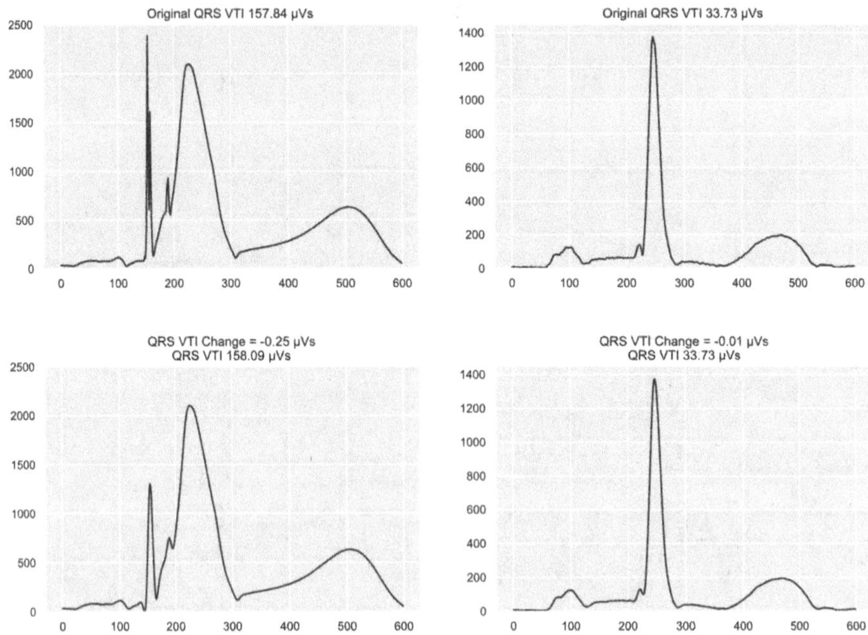

Fig. 14 Same two examples with *150 Hz Butterworth low pass filter* on a cardiac resynchronization therapy (CRT) paced and a non-paced (control) RMS ECG signal

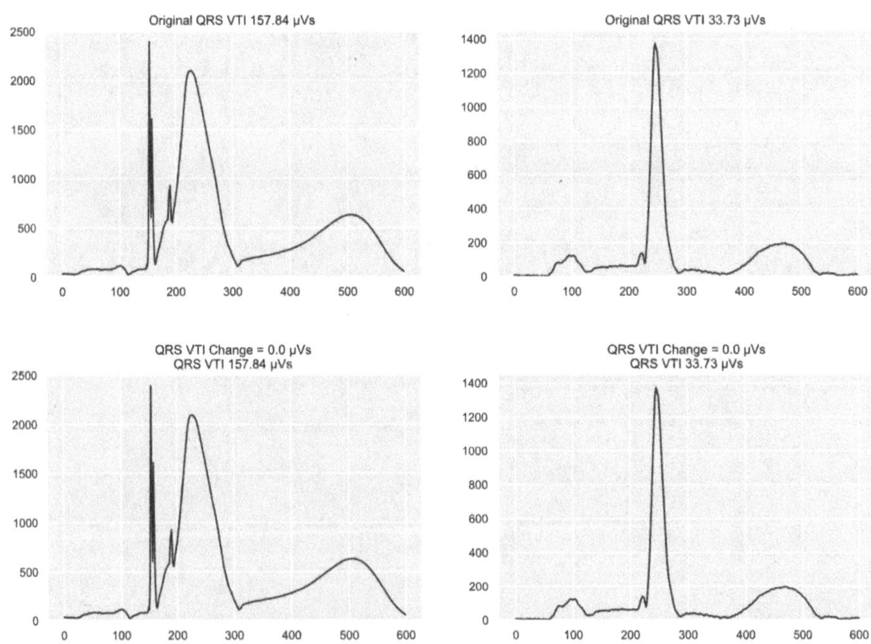

Fig. 15 Same two examples with *Whitaker and Hayes filter* on a cardiac resynchronization therapy (CRT) paced and a non-paced (control) RMS ECG signal

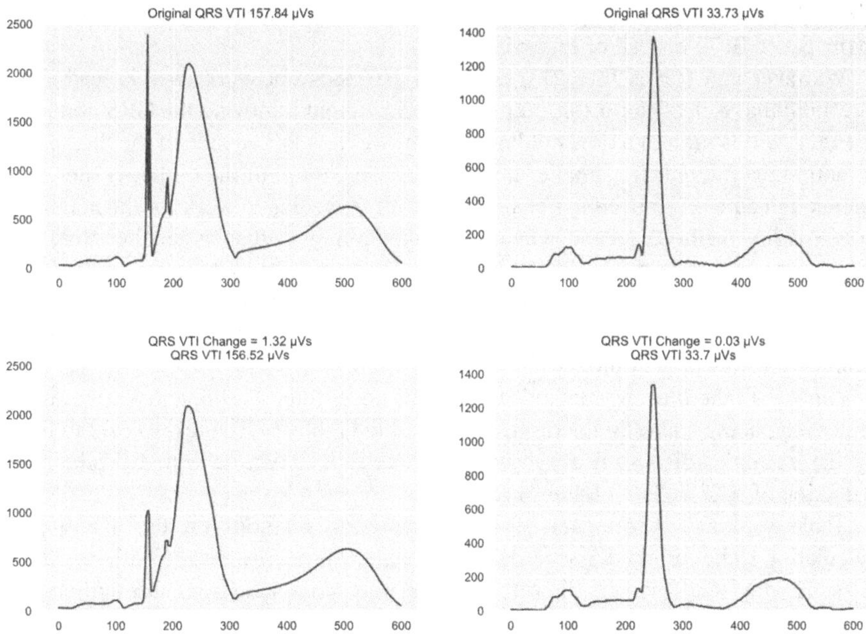

Fig. 16 Same two examples with *Whitaker and Hayes followed by median filter* on a cardiac resynchronization therapy (CRT) paced and a non-paced (control) RMS ECG signal

for the paced ECG but completely removes the QRS complex for the non-paced ECG. It also slightly alters the P wave in the paced ECG which is not favorable.

The LoG filter (Fig. 10) does the third best at removing the outliers, but it also changes the morphology of the QRS complexes. There is a data shift leftward of the second outlier. It also adds some area to the first outlier as it combines the two thin spikes into one shorter but thicker spike. We saw this effect across the board with LoG and not just the difficult case examples as can be seen in Fig. 21.

The Butterworth filters (Figs. 11, 12, 13, and 14) have mixed results. The 60 Hz cutoff frequency (Fig. 11) suffers the same problem as LoG. It shortens the two thin outliers at the start of the QRS complex, but it combines them into one even thicker outlier that adds area to the outlier. It does fully remove the second smaller outlier, which is the only filter to completely smooth that outlier out, but it also shifts the data to the left again like LoG. We can see that it also changes the end of the QRS complex and the P wave before the QRS complex. The same holds true for the non-paced ECG. It greatly reduces the amplitude of the QRS complex and removes the physiological high-frequency components from the QRS morphology. It also smooths out the P wave and the noise surrounding the QRS complex. As we use higher and higher low-pass cutoffs we get worse results in removing the pacing spikes but maintain the integrity of the QRS complex better. The 90 Hz cutoff (Fig. 12) is reasonably balanced. It barely changes the P wave and QRS complex in both the paced and non-paced. It adds width to the first outlier while reducing amplitude.

The 120 Hz and 150 Hz (Figs. 13 and 14 respectively) cutoff frequencies add area to the paced ECG instead of removing area.

Whitaker and Hayes filter (Figs. 15 and 16) does not work on this lead. The threshold that is needed for this outlier to work without removing the QRS complex is 1150. At this high of a threshold none of the outliers fall outside of the threshold, so nothing is filtered. If a smaller threshold is used, more of the outlier is removed but enough data is removed to not allow the rolling median to work for the neighbor interpolation method. As the window for the rolling median is smaller than the outlier and it throws back an error as no data is present. When we applied the median filter after the Whitaker and Hayes filter, it achieved the same results as just the median filter (Fig. 15). This demonstrates the need for a dynamic filter to be able to precisely target outliers.

Among all the filtering methods tested, our novel filter was the most effective at removing pacing spikes in the discussed example (Table 2). The results exemplified by the examples discussed above hold true across our dataset with % spike area reduction of 99.6 ± 8.03 (Table 3).

Table 4 shows the impact of various filtering methods on the $VTI_{QRS\text{-}3D}$ calculation. The original paced ECG average $VTI_{QRS\text{-}3D}$ was 67.87 ± 32.73 μVs. Hampel and median filtering removes the most area from the outliers on average, 67.68 ± 32.65 μVs and 67.67 ± 32.66 μVs, respectively. LoG is third at 67.87 ± 32.73 μVs. The Whitaker and Hayes filter did not remove any area without the median filter being implemented. This is due to the fact that the threshold had to be higher for these types of patients as the 90 ECGs we used were difficult cases. Whitaker and Hayes's algorithm does work on easier samples but still not as well as the novel filter (Fig. 18a–d). The Butterworth filters had insignificant change at scale except 60 Hz which actually added more area on average, 67.98 ± 32.76 μVs, and gave a worse signal back than the original paced signal. All of these signals preformed worse than the novel filter at 67.2 ± 32.5 μVs $VTI_{QRS\text{-}3D}$.

The average non-paced $VTI_{QRS\text{-}3D}$ was 41.79 ± 10.43 μVs. Hampel preformed the worst by far on non-paced ECGs at 26.73 ± 13.52 μVs. This is mainly due to the fact that Hampel filters are overly sensitive to high frequency data and deletes the QRS complex in most of the non-paced ECG signals. The next worse were Butterworth filters. At every cutoff frequency, they added area to the signal. The two best filters for non-paced ECGs are the median filter at 41.68 ± 10.4 μVs and LoG filter at 41.76 ± 10.43 μVs. The LoG and median filter removed noise from the signal while barely altering the original QRS complex. The median filter removed more noise from the signal though which is part of the reason why the overall $VTI_{QRS\text{-}3D}$ is lower for the median filter. Whitaker and Hayes and our novel filter did not change the non-paced ECGs at all until median filtering was applied. For the Whitaker and Hayes's method, this was due to the threshold being abnormally high. If we selected a smaller threshold more of the QRS complex would have been deleted much like the Hampel filter.

These results can be shown even more clearly from Table 2. This table shows the adjusted area reduction by each filter on the hardest leads from Figs. 8, 9, 10, 11, 12, 13, 14, 15, and 16. The original area of the first spike was reduced by 2385

Table 2 Comparing removed area (voltage-time-integral) of pacing spike outliers on the RMS ECG example shown in Figs. 7, 8, 9, 10, 11, 12, 13, 14, 15, and 16 using different filtering methods (n = 1). Negative values for the % removed here mean that area was added to the pacing spike (i.e. the outlier got bigger). Optimal value would be 100% removal

					Butterworth low pass				Novel filter	
Spike area[a]	Original data	Hampel	LoG	Median	60 Hz	90 Hz	120 Hz	150 Hz	Step 1 (outlier)	+Step 2 (median)
First spike (nVs)	10,048	3284	9747	7067	8363	10,080	10,569	10,539	−192	−907
% removed[b]	–	67	3	30	17	−0.3	−5	−5	102	109
Second spike (nVs)	391	391	265	74	−277	201	297	415	391	−16
% removed[b]	–	0	32	81	171	49	24	−6	0	104

LoG Laplace of Gaussian

[a] Area traced by the pacing spike relative to a straight line connecting the physiological signal before and after the spike

[b] Compared to original data

Table 3 Comparing average removed area (voltage-time-integral) of pacing spike outliers on the RMS ECG signal in 90 cardiac resynchronization therapy (CRT) paced ECGs using different filtering methods (n = 90). Negative values for the % removed here mean that area was added to the pacing spike (i.e. the outlier got bigger). Optimal value would be 100% removal

				Butterworth low pass				Novel filter
Spike area[a]	Hampel	LoG	Median	60 Hz	90 Hz	120 Hz	150 Hz	
% removed[b] (mean ± S.D.)	75.8 ± 19.6	7.4 ± 4.62	27.7 ± 6.86	17.9 ± 8.08	7.4 ± 3.81	−1.5 ± 2.37	−2.5 ± 1.84	99.6 ± 8.03

LoG Laplace of Gaussian

[a] Area traced by the pacing spike relative to a straight line connecting the physiological signal before and after the spike

[b] Compared to original data

Table 4 Comparing average QRS 3D-voltage-time-integral ($VTI_{QRS\text{-}3D}$) from RMS ECG leads using different filtering methods. Optimal values for non-paced would be a P-value of 1. Optimal values for paced would be a P-value <0.001

$VTI_{QRS\text{-}3D}$ (mean ± S.D.)	Original data	Hampel	LoG	Median	Butterworth low pass				Whitaker and Hayes	Novel filter
					60 Hz	90 Hz	120 Hz	150 Hz		
Non-paced ECGs (n = 90)	41.79 ± 10.43	26.73 ± 13.52	41.76 ± 10.43	41.68 ± 10.4	41.83 ± 10.42	41.81 ± 10.44	41.81 ± 10.44	41.8 ± 10.43	41.68 ± 10.4	41.4 ± 10.35
P-value[a]	–	1.6e-22	1.8e-14	1.4e-11	0.036	0.0014	1.5e-7	8.7e-7	1.4e-11	0.67
CRT paced ECGs (n = 90)	67.87 ± 32.73	67.68 ± 32.65	67.87 ± 32.73	67.67 ± 32.66	67.98 ± 32.76	67.91 ± 32.75	67.9 ± 32.74	67.9 ± 32.73	67.67 ± 32.66	67.2 ± 32.52
P-value[a]	–	0.0056	0.071	1.1e-11	0.017	0.55	0.71	0.92	1.1e-11	1.2e-9

CRT cardiac resynchronization therapy; *LoG* Laplace of Gaussian; $VTI_{QRS\text{-}3D}$ QRS 3D-voltage-time-integral

[a] T-test comparing to original data

to account for the area below the curve under the outlier that would normally exist anyway. The original area of the second spike was reduced by 6600 for the same reason. The original data in this case was 10,047.9 μVs and 390.5 μVs for the first and second spikes. The Hampel filter was able to reduce 67.3% of the area of the first spike while not filtering the second spike at all. This was the best result from all the filters other than the novel filter. The next best result was from the median filter which was able to filter out 29.7% of the area of the first spike and 81% of the second spike. LoG was third best at 3% and 32.3% for the first and second spikes. This shows that while the amplitude of the spike was greatly decreased, the overall area remained mostly the same as it widened the outlier. All of the Butterworth filters did very poorly. Only the 60 Hz did not add area to the first spike, but it morphed the physiology of the QRS complex enough to make the area removed 170.9%. We want a result as close to 100% as possible and going over too much is just as bad as not changing at all. The Whitaker and Hayes filter was omitted on this table as it did not change at all. The novel filter preformed the best with both steps on the first spike and the best with the second step focused median filter on the second spike. The final reduction in area was 109% and 104.2%. This is as close to perfect as we could get without fine tuning a filter for this specific ECG.

This demonstrates the need for the two-step filter and how just one filter does not fully filter out outliers while also keeping the non-outlier data intact. The novel filter is able to successfully filter out all outliers on every ECG we have without adjusting the non-paced ECGs other than smoothing out noise. It is strong in every situation where each of the above filters are at their best while also being strong when the other filters are not. The novel filter can also be applied at a wide variety of amplitudes and heart conditions.

Figure 17a–f show the novel filter working on extremely large pacing spikes compared to Whitaker and Hayes' method. The amount of outlier left behind by the Whitaker and Hayes' method is still more than enough to invalidate any regression, distance, or area calculation done on these ECGs. This shows the limitation of just a median filter. It works well with very noisy data and even small amplitude outliers, but for the massive outliers that are fairly common among CRT patients it no longer works. The novel filter on the other hand is able to either completely remove the outliers or remove the overwhelming major of its area. Figure 17f shows that the filter can remove both small and large outliers in the same signal. Figure 18a-c show that the novel filter also works very well on low amplitude outliers. This is most clear in Fig. 18a which has three outliers that are all smaller than the QRS complex by a significant amount and yet they are still completely removed. Figure 18d-f show the normal amplitude range of outliers on ECGs with patients that have narrow QRS complexes. Normally in this situation it is hard to filter out the outliers because the QRS complex has a similar modified Z-score as the outliers. We can see that the novel filter is able to filter out these outliers while not augmenting any of the QRS complex even when the QRS complex has a larger amplitude jump than the outlier such as in Fig. 18d.

Figures 19, 20, 21, and 22 are more examples of how the other filters we tested compare to the novel filter on non-RMS ECG signal data. We used a different lead

a

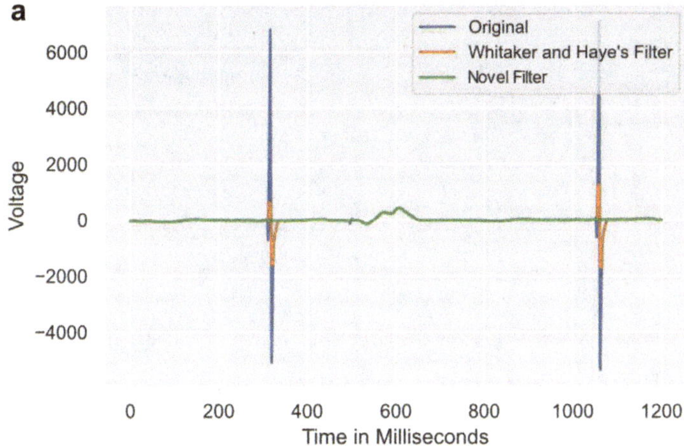

b

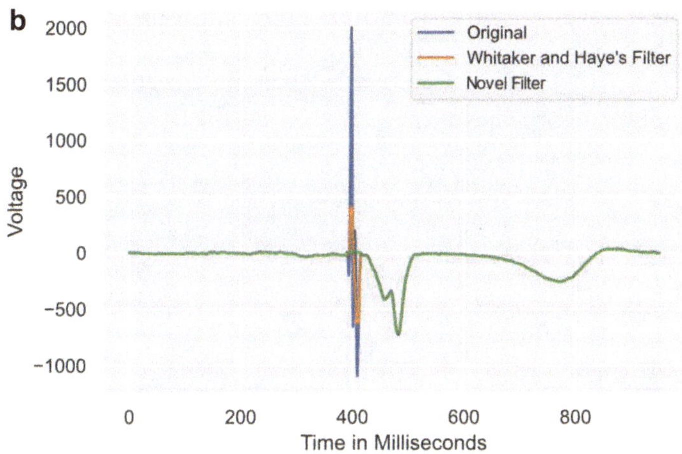

Fig. 17 (**a**) An example comparing the *novel* filter with *Whitaker and Hayes* filter on large amplitude outliers on lead V1. The novel filter can deal with outliers of any size and frequency without the need of extreme fine tuning. (**b**) Another example comparing the *novel* filter with *Whitaker and Hayes* filter on large amplitude outliers on lead V1. This is a very wide and tall outlier and the filter is able to deal with it without distorting the physiological signal. (**c**) Another example comparing the *novel* filter with *Whitaker and Hayes* filter on large amplitude outliers on lead V1. (**d**) Another example comparing the *novel* filter with *Whitaker and Hayes* filter on large amplitude outliers on lead V1. (**e**) An example comparing the *novel* filter with *Whitaker and Hayes* filter on large amplitude outliers on lead V3. This is a case where the hyperbolic cosine function doesn't interpolate the signal very well as can be seen from the sharp deflection of the signal at the Q onset. In this case a cubic spline would be better to interpolate the signal. (**f**) An example comparing the *novel* filter with *Whitaker and Hayes* filter on large amplitude outliers on lead V2. This is a case where the filter couldn't completely delete the outlier in front of the QRS complex. This is due to the QRS complex having a similar Z-score to that part of the outlier. So, when the deletion happens any data point close to the QRS complex will be left behind. We can see that the outlier was still greatly diminished compared to Whitaker and Hayes' filter, but more precise fine tuning would be needed to completely filter out this example

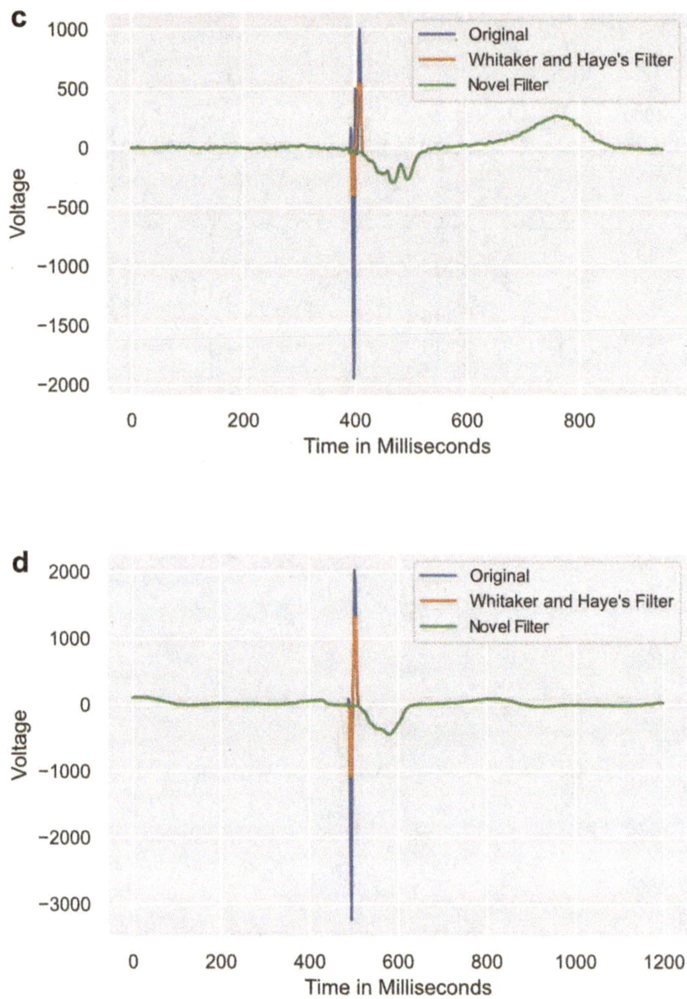

Fig. 17 (continued)

for the Butterworth filters to better show how the filters compare as it was not easy to see with the lead used on the Hampel, LoG, and median filters. Again, we see the same results with one big change. This lead was one we found in which the Hampel filter did not perform as well as the others on the paced ECGs. None of the three filters preform as well as the novel filter. The median was actually the best in this case which holds true from what we saw in Table 2. It goes back and forth with median or Hampel being the best on paced and median being the best on non-paced ECGs. The Butterworth filters also were consistent on these leads. 60 Hz causes the amplitude of the outlier to be much smaller, but the outlier widens and the QRS

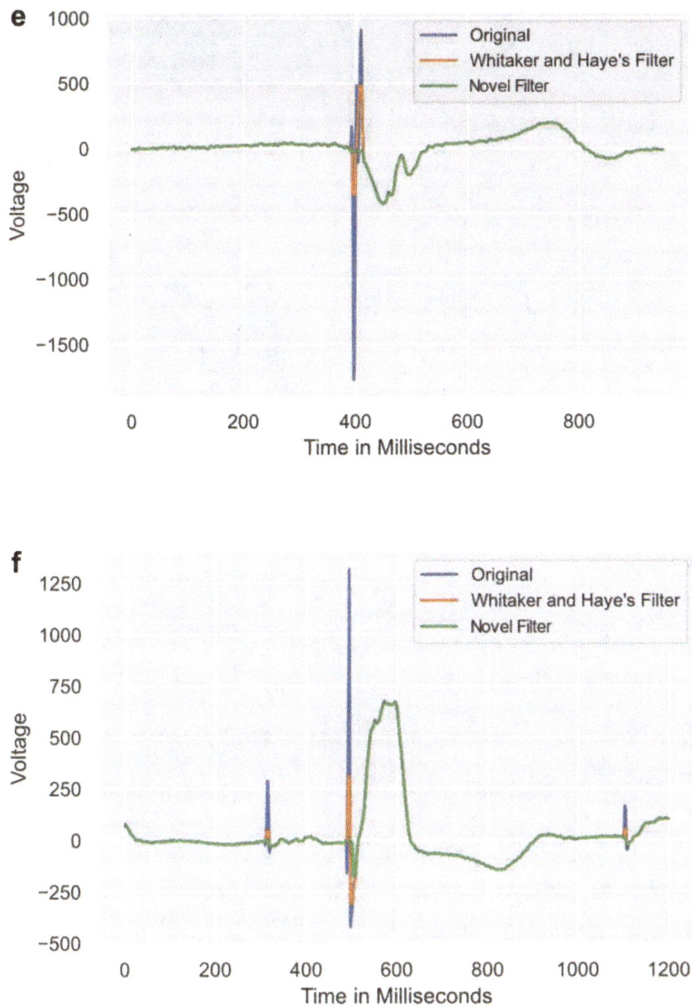

Fig. 17 (continued)

complex is deformed. While 150 Hz causes a minor reduction in outlier amplitude while not changing much of the physiological QRS complex signal.

Figures 23, 24, 25, and 26 are examples of the filters on a very narrow non-paced ECG. The results are as expected. Hampel completely filters out the QRS complex. Median and LoG both filter out perfectly all the noise in the signal while slightly diminishing the QRS complex with the median being the best on the non-paced data. All the Butterworth filters slightly deform the QRS complex which is important as there is so little data in the QRS complex as it is so narrow that all data needs to be as unchanged as possible.

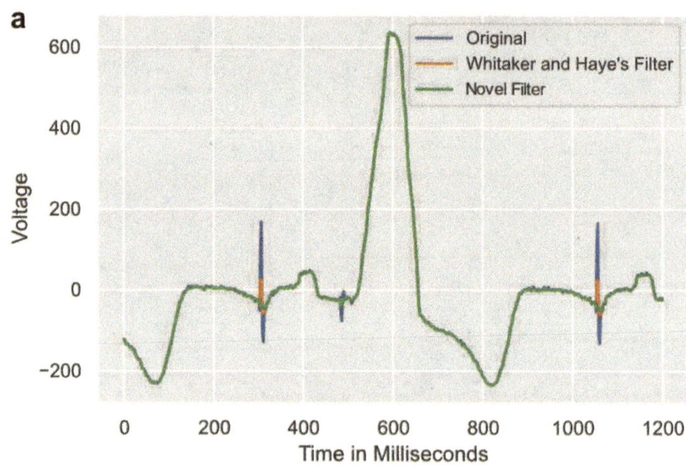

Fig. 18 (**a**) An example comparing the *novel* filter with *Whitaker and Hayes* filter on small amplitude outliers on lead V2. (**b**) An example comparing the *novel* filter with *Whitaker and Hayes* filter on small amplitude outliers on lead II. The novel filter can even filter out similar frequencies and voltages as can be seen in this example. (**c**) An example comparing the *novel* filter with *Whitaker and Hayes* filter on small amplitude outliers on lead I. (**d**) Another example comparing the *novel* filter with *Whitaker and Hayes* filter on normal amplitude outliers on lead I. This example shows that the filter can remove outliers that are similar shape and smaller voltage compared to the QRS complex without fine tuning. (**e**) An example comparing the *novel* filter with *Whitaker and Hayes* filter on normal amplitude outliers on lead V6. (**f**) An example comparing the *novel* filter with *Whitaker and Hayes* filter on normal amplitude outliers on lead V4

We have subsequently applied our novel filtering algorithm to a large set of both CRT paced and non-paced (over 10,000 each) respectively. The first-step outlier

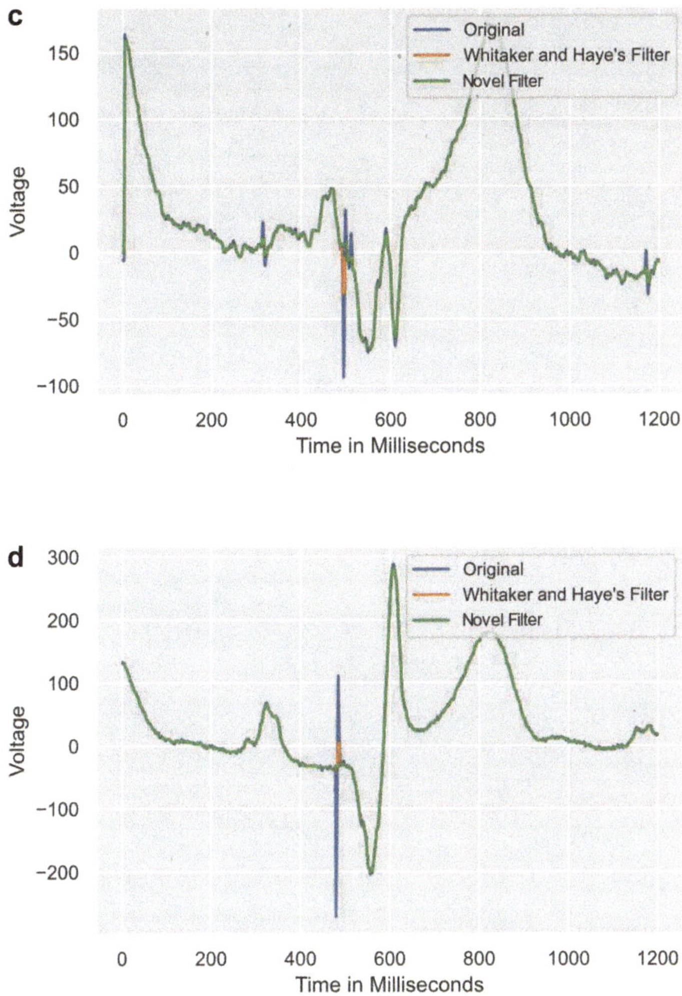

Fig. 18 (continued)

algorithm was very robust in cleanly removing the large problematic pacing spikes, though not infrequently smaller pacing spikes were not picked up at the first step. These were however effectively tackled by the second-step median filter. On the other hand, for rare normal non-paced ECGs (approximately 20–30 ECG leads out of 10,000) with sharp QRS complexes at notably elevated heart rates, the algorithm erroneously detected the sharp peak of QRS complex as outlier. This was however appropriately flagged as an erroneous truncation of the physiological signal at our algorithm's last verification step, and the filter was automatically reverted. The cases in which our filter struggles are fast, sharp non-paced ECGs as mentioned above and

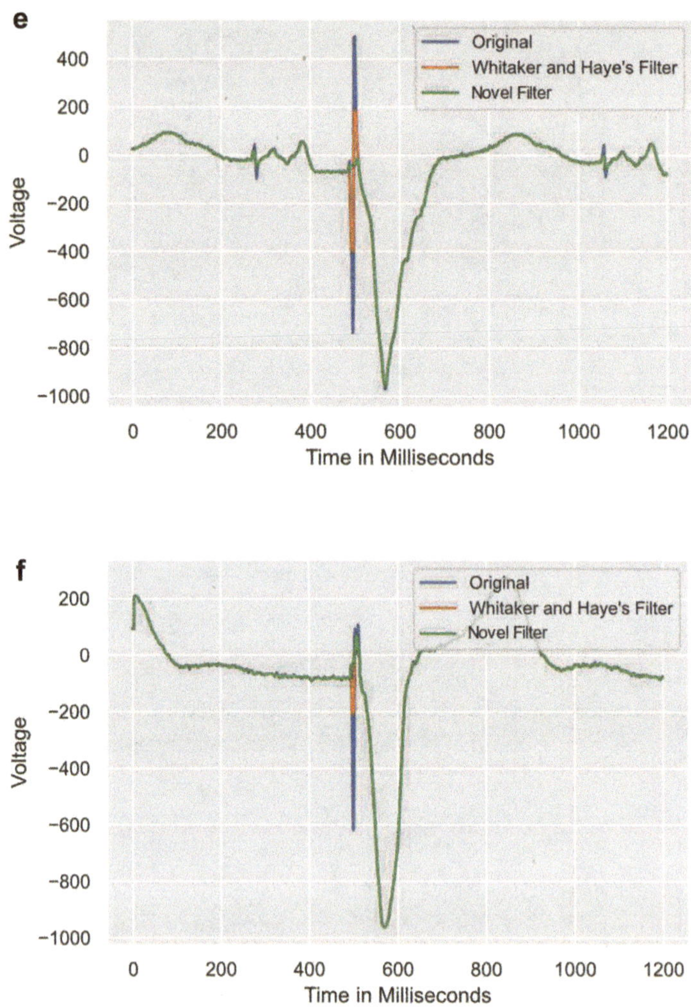

Fig. 18 (continued)

outliers located directly near the peak of the QRS complex. Both are rare, and most ECGs will be filtered successfully.

This filtering process allows us to dynamically filter all outliers with extreme precision. This also allows for near instantaneous processing at 7.53 ms per lead averaged over 4632 leads (time was taken on a desktop PC with a Ryzen 7 1700X CPU and 16 GB of 2400 Hz DDR4 RAM).

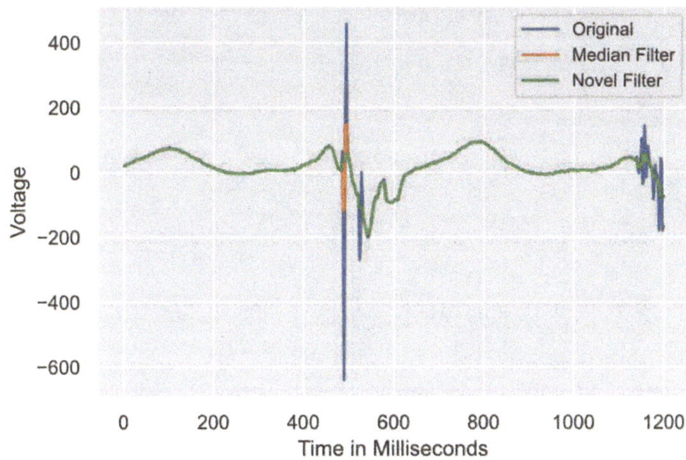

Fig. 19 A cardiac resynchronization therapy (CRT) paced example comparing *novel* filter with *median* filter on lead I. The novel filter was able to remove both of the outliers and smooth out the noise at the end of the signal

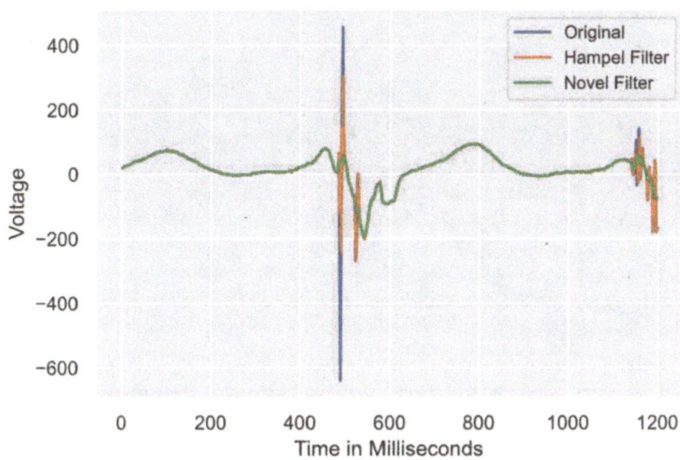

Fig. 20 Same CRT paced ECG comparing *novel* filter with *Hampel* filter on lead I

4 Summary

We present a new dynamic filter to process spike outliers that improves upon the Whitaker and Hayes's despiking algorithm [10] and apply it to ECG data. The outlier detection is done using the modified Z-score of detrended data. The filter interpolates the new signal from the gap generated from deleting data above the dynamic threshold. It then applies a median filter to smooth out the remaining noise.

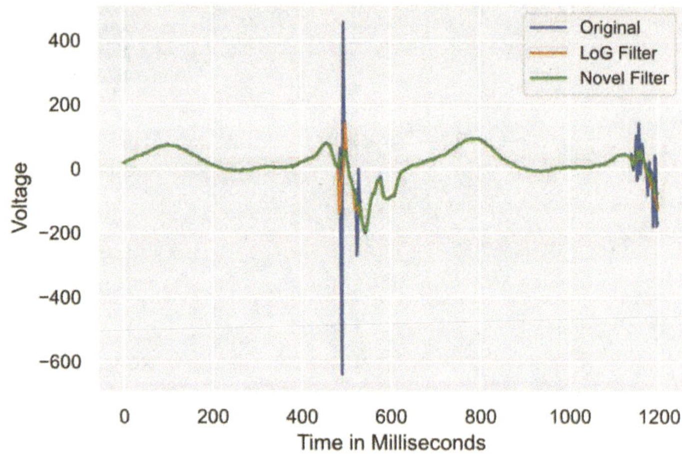

Fig. 21 Same CRT paced ECG comparing *novel* filter with *Laplace of Gaussian (LoG)* filter on lead I

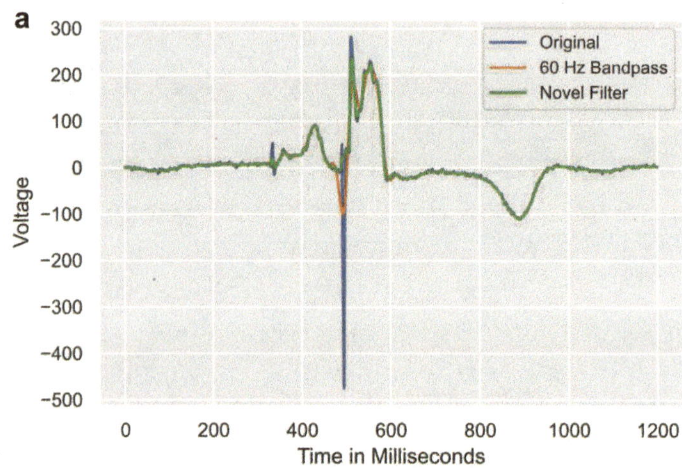

Fig. 22 (**a**) A cardiac resynchronization therapy (CRT) paced example comparing *novel* filter with *60 Hz Butterworth low pass* filter on lead I. We can see that 60 Hz removes the most amount of the outlier, but it also distorts the physiological signal in a way that the novel filter does not. (**b**) Same paced ECG comparing *novel* filter with *90 Hz Butterworth low pass* filter on lead I. (**c**) Same paced ECG comparing *novel* filter with *120 Hz Butterworth low pass* filter on lead I. (**d**) Same paced ECG comparing *novel* filter with *150 Hz Butterworth low pass* filter on lead I

The novel filtering is very effective and reduces the pacing spike artifact area on average by 99.63% compared to unfiltered paced ECGs. Of the other filters tested, Hampel was the second best for paced ECGs at 75.8%, median filtering was third at 27.7%, 60 Hz Butterworth was fourth at 17.9% (but that included a good amount

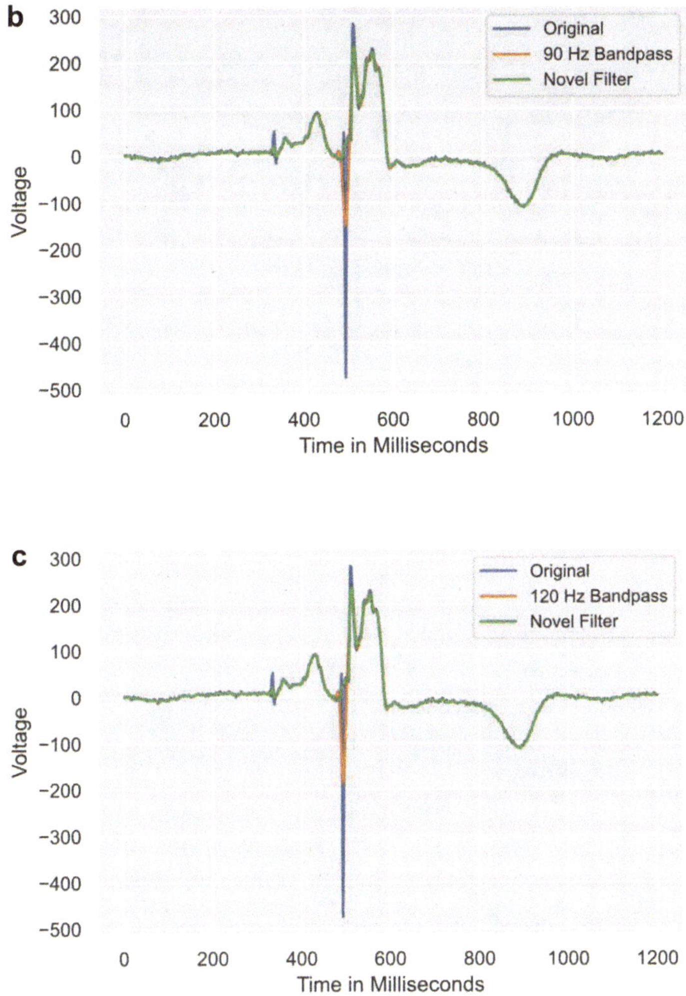

Fig. 22 (continued)

of QRS complex augmentation), LoG was fifth at 7.4%. Higher cut off Butterworth filters were less effective, 90 Hz reduced area only 3.8%, while 120 Hz at −1.5% and 150 Hz at −2.5% both added area to the spike artifacts (Table 3).

The filtering has been demonstrated to be robust and reliable on 12 lead ECG data in many patients spanning a variety of cardiovascular conditions. This filter is computationally inexpensive, fast (7.53 ms per lead, on AMD Ryzen 7 1700x CPU), and can be applied on any platform. This filter can also be applied for any type of signal or time series data and can be applied generally across domains with only tuning of the percentile of Z-scores and the flat value of the filter and changing the starting point of the scan.

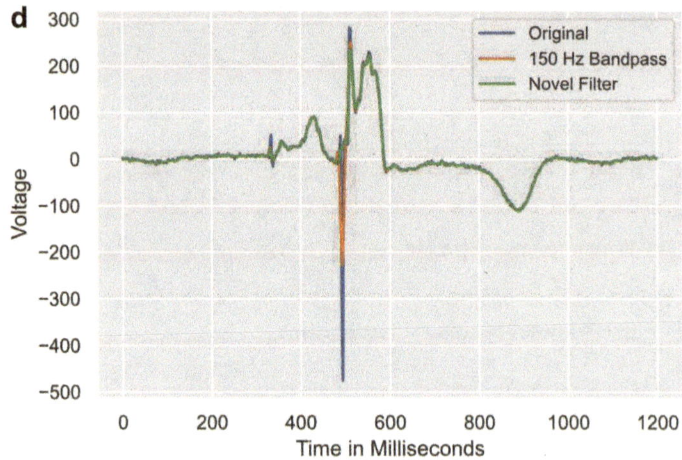

Fig. 22 (continued)

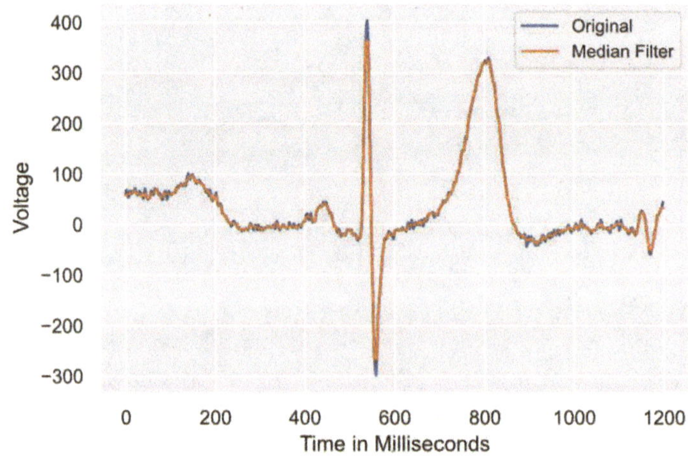

Fig. 23 An example of *median* filter applied to a non-paced ECG lead II. This outlier does very well for non-paced ECG even with narrow QRS complexes

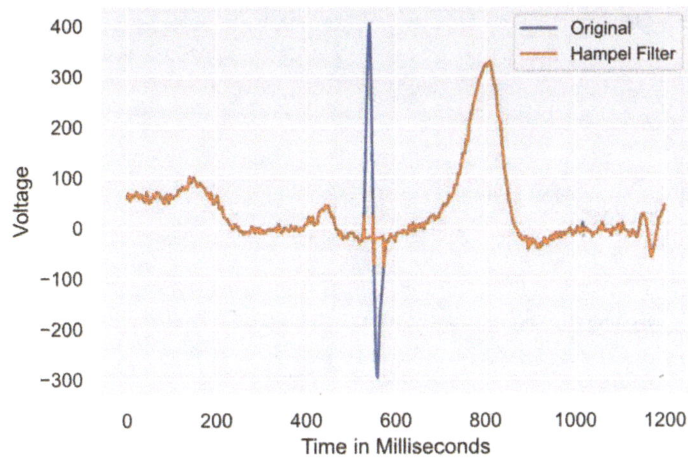

Fig. 24 An example of *Hampel* filter applied to the same non-paced ECG lead II. The QRS complex signal is destroyed

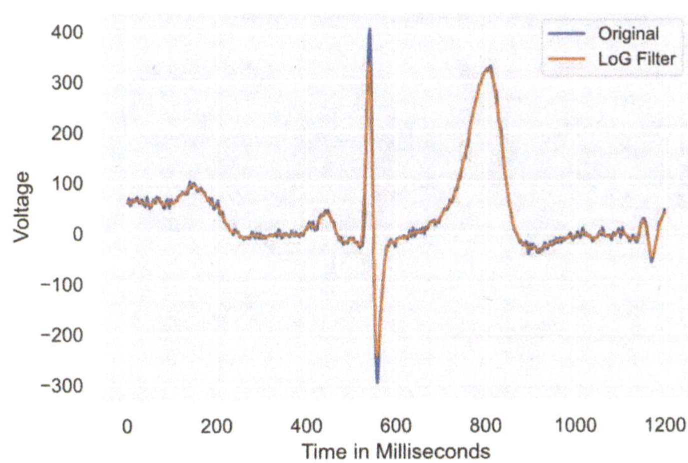

Fig. 25 An example of *Laplace of Gaussian (LoG)* filter applied to the same non-paced ECG lead II. Slightly worse than median filtering but still better than most methods

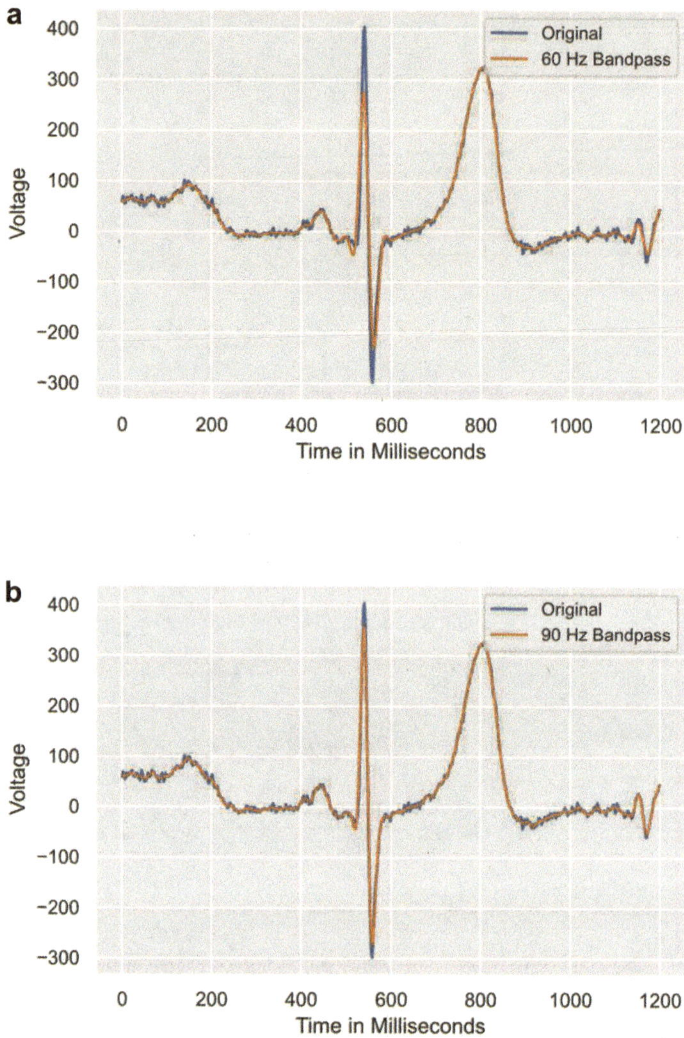

Fig. 26 (**a**) An example of 60 Hz Butterworth low pass filter applied to the same non-paced ECG lead II. 60 Hz works well for paced ECG but not nearly as well for non-paced. The signal is also distorted before the QRS complex. (**b**) An example of 90 Hz Butterworth low pass filter applied to the same non-paced ECG lead II. (**c**) An example of 120 Hz Butterworth low pass filter applied to the same non-paced ECG lead II. (**d**) An example of 150 Hz Butterworth low pass filter applied to the same non-paced ECG lead II. 150 Hz works as well as median filtering on non-paced ECG but not as well for outliers

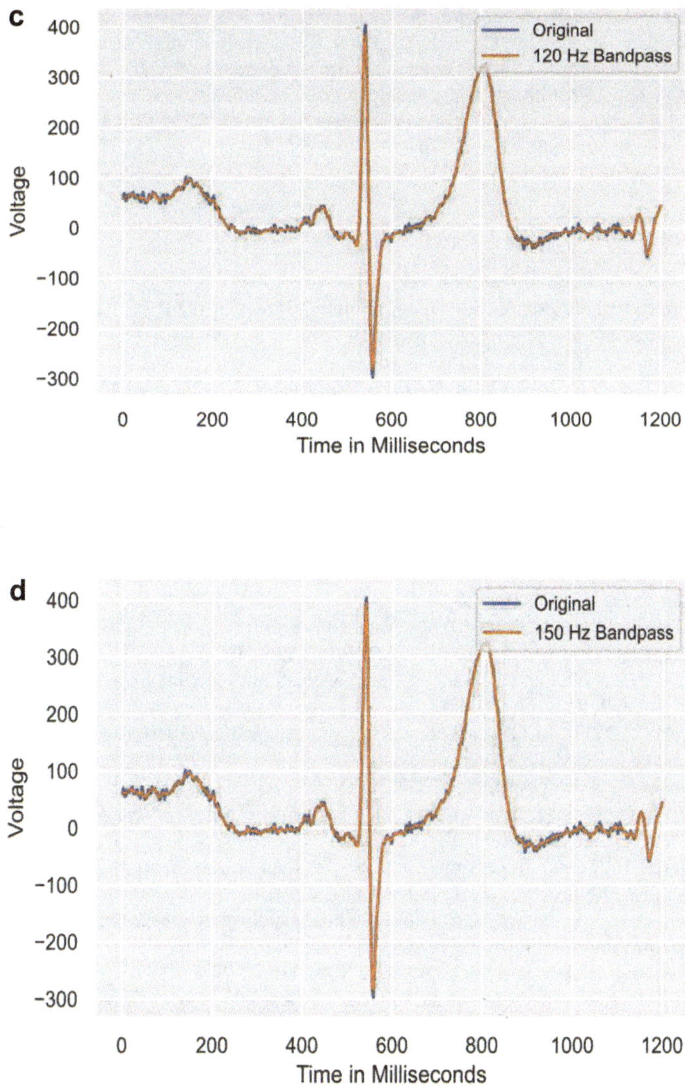

Fig. 26 (continued)

Acknowledgments Research reported in this publication was supported by The University of Kansas and University of Kansas Medical Center Research Institute. The content is solely the responsibility of the authors and does not necessarily represent the official views of The University of Kansas. Any opinions, findings, and conclusions or recommendations expressed in this material are those of the authors and do not necessarily reflect the views of The University of Kansas.

References

1. Plesinger, F., van Stipdonk, A. M. W., Smisek, R., et al. (2019). Fully automated QRS area measurement for predicting response to cardiac resynchronization therapy. *Journal of Electrocardiology, 63*, 159–163.
2. Noheria, A., Sodhi, S., & Orme, G. J. (2019). The evolving role of electrocardiography in cardiac resynchronization therapy. *Current Treatment Options in Cardiovascular Medicine, 21*, 1–14.
3. Okafor, O., et al. (2019). Changes in QRS area and QRS duration after cardiac resynchronization therapy predict cardiac mortality, heart failure hospitalizations, and ventricular arrhythmias. *Journal of the American Heart Association, 8*(21), e013539.
4. De Pooter, J., et al. (2017). Biventricular paced QRS area predicts acute hemodynamic CRT response better than QRS duration or QRS amplitudes. *Journal of Cardiovascular Electrophysiology, 28*(2), 192–200.
5. Jaffe, L. M., & Morin, D. P. (2014). Cardiac resynchronization therapy: History, present status, and future directions. *The Ochsner Journal, 14*(4), 596–607.
6. Li, K., Du, N., & Zhang, A. (2012). Detecting ECG abnormalities via Transductive transfer learning. *ACM-BCB, 2012*, 210–217.
7. Sun, Y., et al. (2002). ECG signal condition by morphological filtering. *Computers in Biology and Medicine, 32*, 564–479.
8. Chandraker, C., & Kowar, M. K. (2012). DENOISING ECG SIGNALS USING ADAPTIVE FILTER ALGORITHM. *International Journal of Soft Computing and Engineering (IJSCE), 2*(1).
9. Kher, R. (2019). Signal processing techniques for removing noise from ECG signals. *Journal of Biomedical Engineering and Research, 3*(101), 1–9.
10. Whitaker, D. A., & Hayes, K. (2018). A simple algorithm for despiking Raman spectra. *Chemometrics and Intelligent Laboratory Systems, 179*, 82–84.
11. Kors, J. A., Van Herpen, G., Sittig, A. C., & Van Bemmel, J. K. (1990). Reconstruction of the Frank vectorcardiogram from standard electrocardiographic leads: Diagnostic comparison of different methods. *European Heart Journal, 11*, 1083–1092.
12. Iglewicz, B., & Hoaglin, D. (1993). *How to detect and handle outliers. The ASQC Basic References in Quality Control: Statistical Techniques* (vol. 16). ISBN 9780873892476.
13. Heckert, N. A., & Filliben, J. J. (2003) *Exploratory data analysis. NIST/SEMATECH e-handbook of statistical methods* (vol. 1; Chap. 1).
14. Bathelt, J. (2018). *Draw a curve connecting two points instead of a straight line*. Stack Overflow. Retrieved from https://stackoverflow.com/questions/30008322/draw-a-curve-connecting-two-points-instead-of-a-straight-line.

Index

I. Obeid et al. (eds.), *Biomedical Sensing and Analysis*,
https://doi.org/10.1007/978-3-030-99383-2